6.13.2023

Amanda

Sending you buckets of love – support – and healing your way –

One day at a time

All my love –
Diana xo

I dedicate this book to my three parents, Papa, Pam and Mom who have continued to remind me of the value of sitting around a dinner table surrounded with the ones I love and a buffet of great food.

"In the twenty-five years or so I served as Executive Chef of the Union Square Café, I had the pleasure to meet and mentor a great many young cooks. Diana Barnett stands out in my memory for her unbridled enthusiasm, diligent application to her work, and irrepressible creativity. I am delighted and proud to see how Diana has responded to her life challenges by creating this book of beautifully photographed, delicious, and healthful tips." - CHEF MICHAEL ROMANO, FORMER EXECUTIVE CHEF OF THE UNION SQUARE CAFÉ

"I have known Diana Barnett for over thirty years, and she continues to amaze me with her unflagging energy and creativity. This book is a perfect example of how she takes what some would consider a negative and turns it into a joyous opportunity to share her positive outlook and natural gifts for cooking and photography. After forty years of a chef's unhealthy habits, I may just have to practice what Diana is preaching!" - CHEF SUSAN SPICER, CHEF/ OWNER BAYONA, MONDO, ROSEDALE

"Diana is an impassioned chef who is evidently using her gifts to make a difference in her health. Her curiosity, kindness, and creativity is an inspiration." - STEFANIE SACKS, MS, CNS, CDN, CULINARY NUTRITIONIST & AUTHOR OF "WHAT THE FORK ARE YOU EATING"

"Chef Di embraces the concept of food as medicine in this powerful and delicious book! Healing others begins with healing thyself. Thank you for sharing your story." - DR. ROBERT GRAHAM, CO-FOUNDER OF FRESHMED

"Eat to live, don't live to eat. The body is the greatest machine known to mankind, and deserves to have the best fuel possible to allow it to run at its optimum performance." - BRYANT JOHNSON, MASTER TRAINER & CREATOR OF RBG WORKOUT

"Diana has been my client for over eight years. When she was diagnosed with diabetes, I focused on building up her muscle mass due to the many benefits. Her drive and determination are admirable and in line with her accomplishment of this beautiful book! I am so proud of her and honored to take this journey alongside her."
- MEL ROBINSON, MASTER TRAINER & AUTHOR OF "FROM FLIPPIN' WEIGHT TO FLIPPING WEIGHTS"

FOREWARD

In writing the foreword to this important book, I hope to give you a small glimpse into the energy field that is Diana Barnett. Let me go back quite a few years to when Diana and I were both working chefs in New York City. I had just launched a small farm-to-table restaurant in Soho called Quilty's. I had my hands more than full with the daily operations as well as trying to be available to food writers and other food world luminaries in my downtime. Our mutual friend, Steven Hall, introduced us. The details are hazy, and I can't remember if we met at Quilty's or elsewhere. But what I do recall is how Diana immediately treated me like a beloved friend, and I was a little confused. "Who is this tall, beautiful woman with the penetrating yet warm brown eyes who seems to know me already?" I didn't trust the energy at that time. I had too many people wanting to "know" me as the chef of a hot new restaurant. However, it started to make sense when I learned Diana herself was a Culinary Institute of America graduate and one of New York City's best chefs at a powerhouse of a restaurant called Time Café.

I can only piece together how we became such good friends by remembering the little moments, and there are so many. Diana never forgot a birthday or a special day of any kind. There was always a call, a card, or a gift. She never forgot where I was in my personal life or what type of drama or blissfully calm seas I was experiencing at the time. I found out from other friends that I was hardly alone—Di kept all of her people in the warm glow of her attention and affection.

Diana was the first person I told I was getting a divorce. I just knew I could trust her with that raw and sad part of me, and she did not disappoint. She was also one of the first people who understood the terrible sense of guilt and helplessness I felt when my son was diagnosed on the autism spectrum at age five. Diana supported my quest to find a way to support his growth in every kind of way through acquiring a deeper knowledge of nutrition. I think it was then that we both recognized our mutual love of food went well beyond the enjoyment of cooking and sharing meals. We knew that good food, thoughtfully prepared was healing, and one of the most profound expressions of love.

It is with real gratitude that I see Diana is turning the laser-like focus she has for others on her own well-being and toward her own healing. In writing and creating this book, she has documented her own journey back to health in a way that will help anyone who follows along. So, count me in! Diana has made it clear she does not see her diabetes as a foe to be conquered, so much as a part of her that needs more love and attention—something Di has spent her life giving to others.

Diana is listening to her body, and her body is saying it is in pain—a deep kind of pain that conventional treatments can't touch. From birth, her body has endured challenges that only the strength of her spirit and the generosity of her heart have been able to absorb and re-direct. It is this remarkable ability Diana has that keeps her going, with tons of credit going to Billy, the love of her life with whom she celebrates life and for whom she stays strong. Self-care helps, and she is continuing on the path to allow that for herself. We should all be on that path, but there are so many cultural messages telling us we are self-involved or self-centered when we say, "Sorry, but no. I can't do X, Y, Z today because I need to take care of myself." But you can start here with Diana as your loving, attentive guide.

Finally, the artist in all of us will no doubt respond to the beauty of Di's photographs and be inspired to jump into our own kitchens and create healing, nourishing, and soul-satisfying meals for ourselves and those we love.

Katy Sparks, Chef and Owner

Katy Sparks Culinary Consulting
"Local, Sustainable, Delicious!"

INTRO

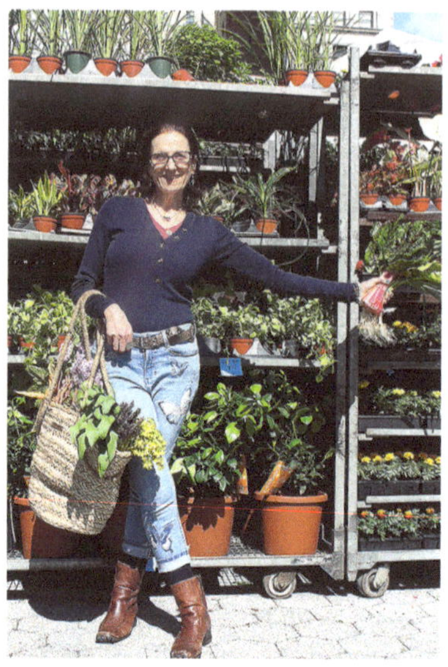

On April 15th, 2018, I walked into my Doctor's office for a regular checkup. After my blood tests came back, the doctor sat me down and explained that my blood sugar was 451 mg, and my A1c levels were 13.7%. She proceeded to tell me I was a diabetic and may possibly have pancreatic cancer. Then the nurse handed me a pretty goodie bag full of needles, strips, and a glucose meter and sent me on my way! To put things into perspective, at that time, I was a relatively healthy person with no family history of diabetes and a chef who knew food. All I could think of was…HOLY CRAP! My life just changed in an instant! Why? How? Now what?

First things first. I do not have pancreatic cancer. The doctor who said I might have it dropped that bomb on me without even making eye contact. She was even typing on her computer when she said it (but that's a whole other book). Second, I decided as a well-trained chef to take my life into my own hands, jump back into the kitchen, and get in tune with my body. After each meal and with each ingredient, I started asking my body questions. I actually checked in with my body and asked how it was feeling and I listened! That is a biggie for me.

I was born in Florence, Italy, so naturally, if you asked me what I would want for my last meal, I'd tell you a huge wheel of Parmigiano-Reggiano, luscious piles of Prosciutto di Parma, and an aromatic bottle of Barolo. Of course, I love pasta. Simply adore it. Did I mention I have a secret love affair with pizza? Oh, and I'm not too shy to admit my mouth waters just thinking of a fresh crusty baguette—right out of the oven—with a chunk of creamy Normandy butter and a delicate sprinkle of pink Himalayan salt. Pure heaven. But here's the thing. I noticed when I indulged in those rich, delectable foods and listened to my body, it wasn't happy with me. My stomach would swell, and I'd joke with my husband, "Look, honey, we're having a baby." Well, of course, you know my protruding belly was not a baby. My gut was crying out for help when the inflammation from eating these types of food stretched and pulled at my insides in unhealthy ways.

Today marks a year of living with diabetes, and I can tell you, my world has changed in profound ways. It's changed in healthy, fulfilling, and satisfying ways, not in the ways I thought it would when I walked out of that "routine checkup" with my diagnosis and my pretty goodie bag. At that point, I think I may have wanted to write a book called, "WTF! How My Diabetes Has Changed My Life." But, I put that on hold. I wanted to explore what I could learn from all this upheaval in my life. My diagnosis taught me more about the condition of my body—mainly my gut—and it was actually not in great shape. I visited many doctors, ran many tests, and tried many different meal plans from Keto to Mediterranean to what I call, Keto-Medo. But for me it came down to this—every day I needed to heal through food, and I am so grateful I learned that. During my holistic healing, I realized it was more than just the food healing me. I healed through food, mind, body, and soul. Tapping into each one of those healing pillars brought me closer to living a fully balanced, healthy lifestyle.

In response to my illness, I created a program called, Healing Fully, Living Freely, which uses the four pillars of healing through food, mind, body, and soul. For me, this program completes the full package of healing and brings me closer to living a healthy daily lifestyle. I use this program to check into the level of satisfaction for each of the four pillars. I then shine a light on the pillar that needs the most attention. This program became the ultimate recipe for healing fully and completely. Today healing fully and living freely is my constant goal, and I work on it every day.

So why this book? I am a photographer as well as a chef, and through my healing process, I have been doing quite a lot of both. A few months ago, I met this really cool eighteen-year-old girl, Hailey Valentine. For any of you General Hospital fans, you will understand why I nearly died when I met her! Her mom named her after one of my favorite soap actor characters. She is an artist herself and worked as a graphic art designer at a local store. When we met, she had just completed her first book on graffiti in Brooklyn. Not only did I love her book, but I also loved her vibe. She was super smart and humble, a little nerdy, and an old soul. I immediately hired her to be my "Millennial Mentor." Before I knew it, we were busy trading ideas and began working on this coffee-table food book full of beautiful photos, introducing twenty-five of the ingredients that had been healing me, each with a Chef Di tip.

Once Hailey became my muse, I went searching for a nutritionist expert. I asked my own nutritionist, Tanya Freirich, who has nine letters of credentials after her name if she would be willing to write the health benefits for my book. Real health benefits. Not the ones we find in our own searches but the solid, up-to-date, proven health benefits fact-checked through the USDA National Nutrient Database, reliable scientific studies, and peer journals. She happily agreed. I created the title of this book, Healthy Food, Happy Me, and built a solid team around it using strong resources.

Through this book, my wish is to share, inspire, and give hope to those who stand outside their own doctor's offices wondering what any type of diagnosis has in store for them, and how all of us can take back a little control—one day at a time.

With gratitude & grace, Diana Barnett

Important Disclaimer: The Information in this book is based on Chef Di's personal experience and research, including third part research where noted. Chef Di is not a doctor. The information in this book has not been evaluated by the Food & Drug Administration, nor is it intended to diagnose, treat, prevent, mitigate, or cure any medical condition. The Information in this book is not a substitute for a one-on-one relationship with a doctor or other qualified healthcare professional.

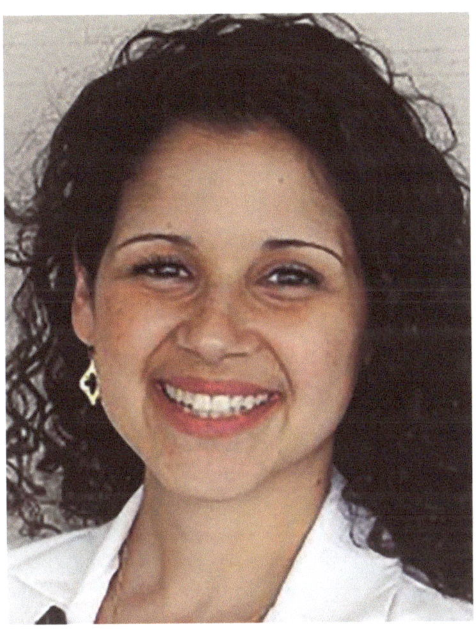

Tanya B. Freirich, MS, RD, CDN, CDE is a Registered Dietitian Nutritionist and Certified Diabetes Educator based in New York City. Tanya shares her passion for nutrition and healing through one-on-one nutrition counseling and group and corporate wellness training. Her expert opinions are found in respected publications such as GQ and AM New York.

Tanya and Diana met professionally through one-on-one nutrition counseling. Since their first appointment together, Diana has applied Tanya's nutrition expertise to take control of her diabetes. "My passion is helping others live their healthiest and happiest lives through dietary and lifestyle changes!"

www.TanyaBNutrition.com

PEACHES

CHEF DI'S TIPS

I adore peaches! The minute these golden beauties are displayed in their lovely symmetrical rows at the Farmer's Market, my mouth and stomach flutter with happy vibes. Of course, as a diabetic, I have to be super careful with the natural sugars in this sweet juicy fruit. Lucky for me, some health studies include peaches as an approved fruit to eat in moderation. As far as eating peaches as a whole, there are so many wonderful options. Plain Jane totally works. Or for a delectable sweet and savory treat, I recommend taking half of a peach, lightly drizzling the top with extra virgin olive oil, a thin slice of prosciutto, a sprig of arugula, and a sprinkle of cracked black pepper. This delightful symphony of aromatic and tangy flavors will transport you to the green rolling hills of Tuscany. If you close your eyes, I may just meet you there, and we can both celebrate this simple yet enchanting combination together.

TANYA'S HEALTH BENEFITS

√ Excellent source of vitamin C - a powerful antioxidant known for promoting healthy skin and immunity.

√ High in potassium - helps maintain healthy blood pressure levels. Ongoing research continues to examine peaches and the possibility that their antioxidants, polyphenols, and other components may be helpful in the prevention of Type 2 Diabetes and obesity by inhibiting certain enzymes in the body.

√ Nectarines and peaches differ by only one gene - that gene controls the relative skin fuzziness!

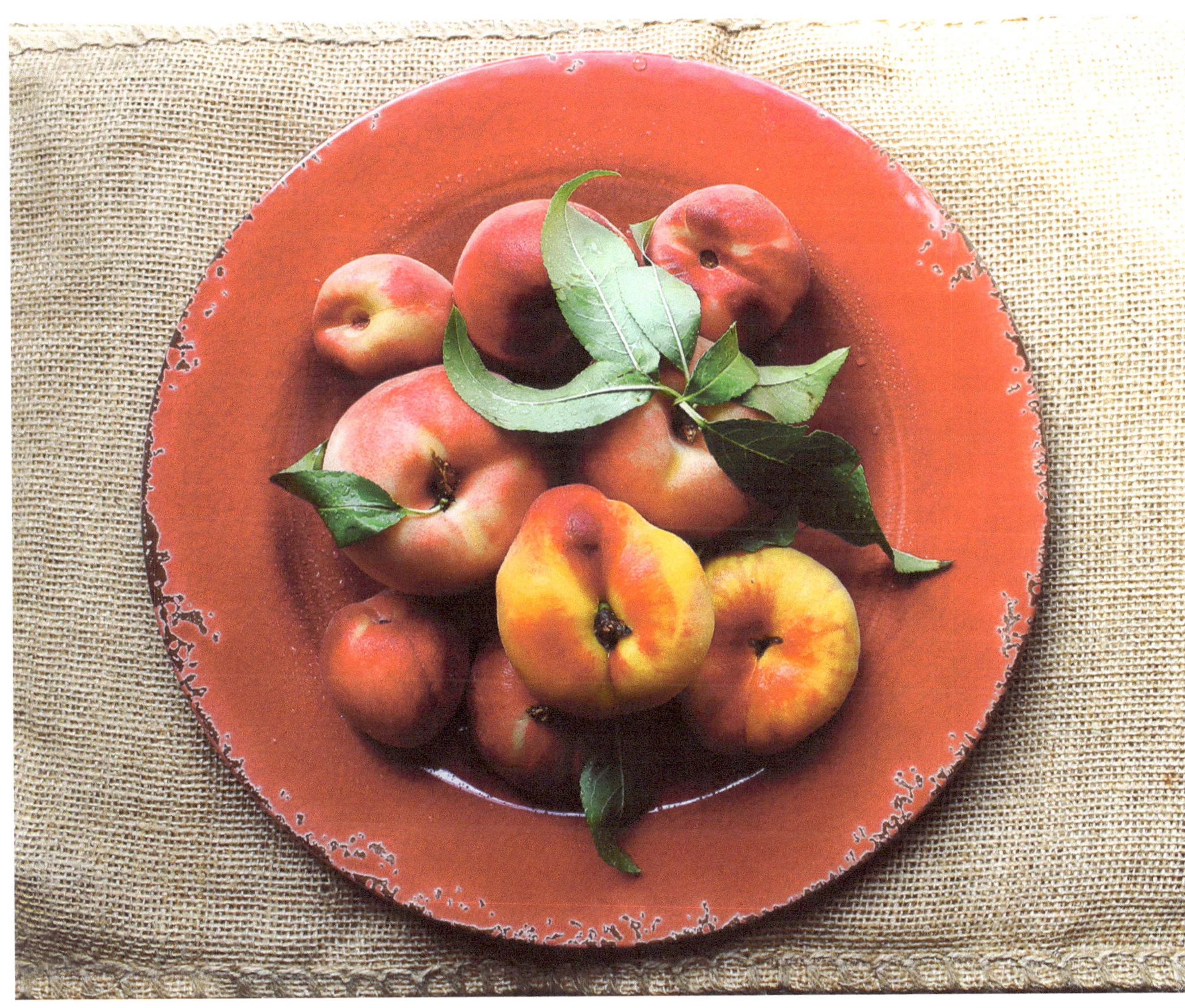

AVOCADOS

CHEF DI'S TIPS

I eat avocados all the time! This green goddess is always good for a simple snack. I also find it is the perfect healthy addition to any entrée or side dish. Adding thick chunky slices of avocado to a bed of mixed greens surrounded by juicy red cherry tomatoes, thinly sliced cucumbers, and purple radishes, with a splash of extra virgin olive oil, lime zest, and sesame seeds are pure perfection to my belly. I will even layer a sliver or two of avocado onto my soft, fluffy scrambled eggs and pieces of chipotle goat cheese. I do find myself tempted to add the smooth buttery texture of an avocado to the occasional fish dish. Imagine sitting at a beachside café, the aroma of salty sea water mixing with the smokiness of a plate of grilled salmon nestled on a bed of roasted red onions. Top it with a few slices of avocado and a sprinkle of black sesame seeds, and you have perfection. Yum!

TANYA'S HEALTH BENEFITS

√ High in potassium - helps lower blood pressure. One half of avocado contains more potassium than a medium banana and has less natural sugar.
√ Technically a fruit, avocados are one the lowest sugar fruits around with only 0.2 grams of sugar per one-half avocado.
√ Excellent source of fiber - helpful in maintaining a healthy digestive system.
√ Keeps your heart healthy - the fat in avocados can lower your total cholesterol number.
√ When combined with a food source of vitamin A, like carrots or tomatoes, avocados can boost your absorption of vitamin A by two to six time.

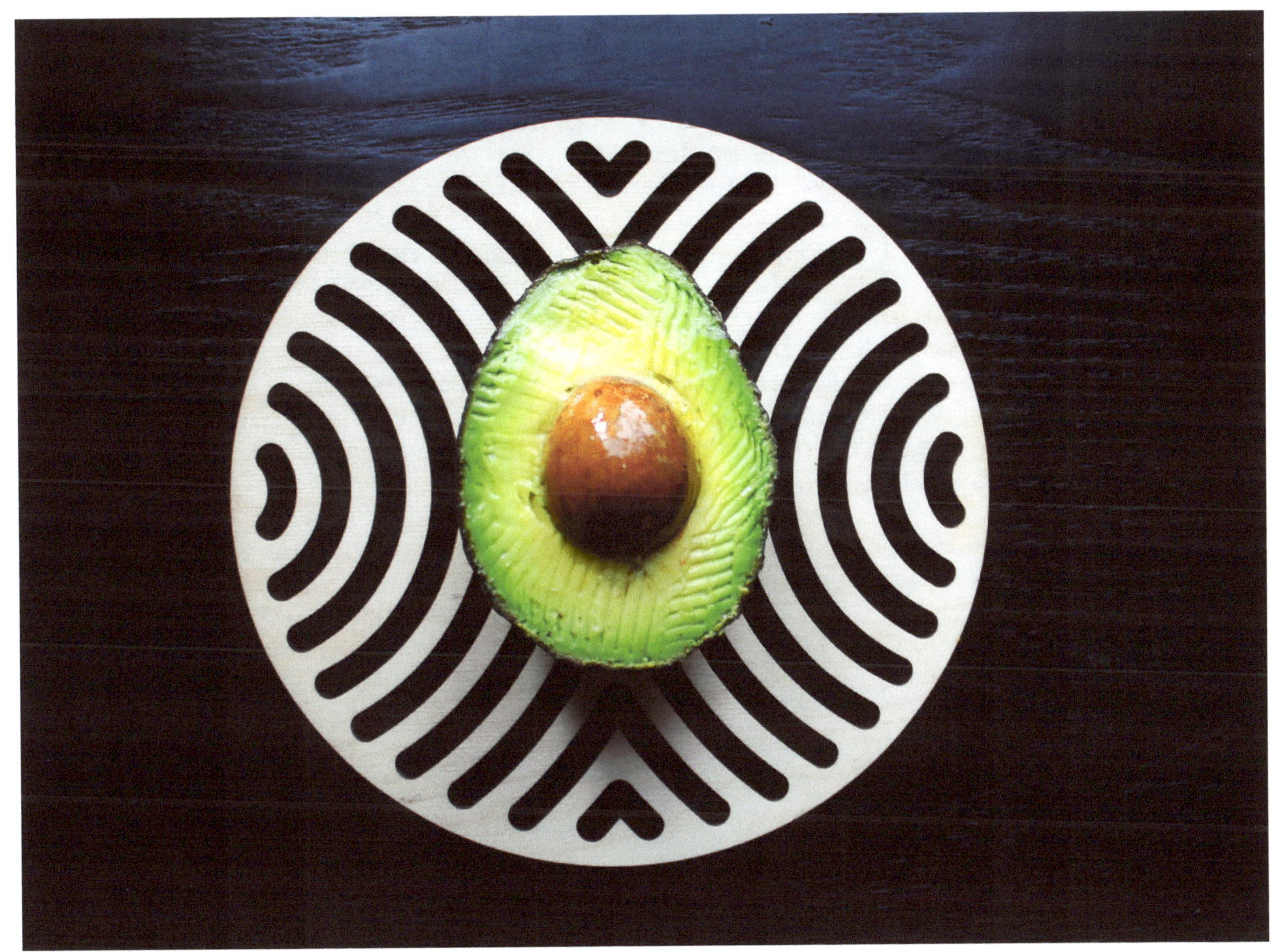

LEMONS & LIMES

CHEF DI'S TIPS

Lemons and limes are staples in my kitchen. I cannot live without them. Years ago, back in New Orleans, my dear friend and mentor Chef Susan Spicer taught me the value of acid in cooking. Chef Spicer explained how acid can create balance in any dish, and indeed it does. A squeeze of tart citrus highlights the best qualities in each individual ingredient's flavor. If you ever taste a particular food on your plate and think to yourself, "Hmm, this is good, but something is missing," I guarantee if you squeeze a little bit of lemon or lime on it, the flavors of each ingredient will be heightened and they will POP!

Sometimes, to enhance my dishes with a little bit of zing, I add citrus zest instead of using the juice. Whenever I sauté a medley of wild mushrooms, I finish it off with zested lemon. I also use a generous twist of lime and a pinch of zest on my roasted chili-herbed-rubbed pork chops. I always add it to my homemade vinaigrettes to not only sharpen each distinct flavor but to add a nice zesty flair. Here's a little secret…lemon and lime zest aren't just for savory dishes. One day while making my turmeric-nut oatmeal, I was inspired by my niece Sophie who told me she adds lemon zest to her oatmeal. Wow! It made my oatmeal dish with all its various flavors truly come alive.

In addition to the cooking benefits, I also wake up every morning and have a glass of water (preferably room temperature) with bursts of fresh-squeezed lemon juice. Citrus acts as nature's alkalizing agent and can not only help flush the digestion system, it can also assist the body with rehydration after the six, seven, or eight hours of fasting while sleeping. Plus, it tastes great and makes me feel fabulous. Lemon and lime—give 'em a squeeze!

TANYA'S HEALTH BENEFITS

√ Only 1 oz. of lemon or lime juice will provide your body with 23% of your daily value of vitamin C.

√ Vitamin C boosts your absorption of iron when combined with a high-iron food.

√ Adding a splash of lemon or lime to spinach will boost it's already generous health benefits.

√ Key limes, in particular, are known to have potent anti-tumor effects and may even help prevent cancer long term.

√ Lemons and limes are the solutions to a debilitating and life-threatening condition called scurvy - a severe vitamin C deficiency that sorely affected the health of sailors during the 1800s. Even today, the British navy requires each of tits ships to have lemons on board.

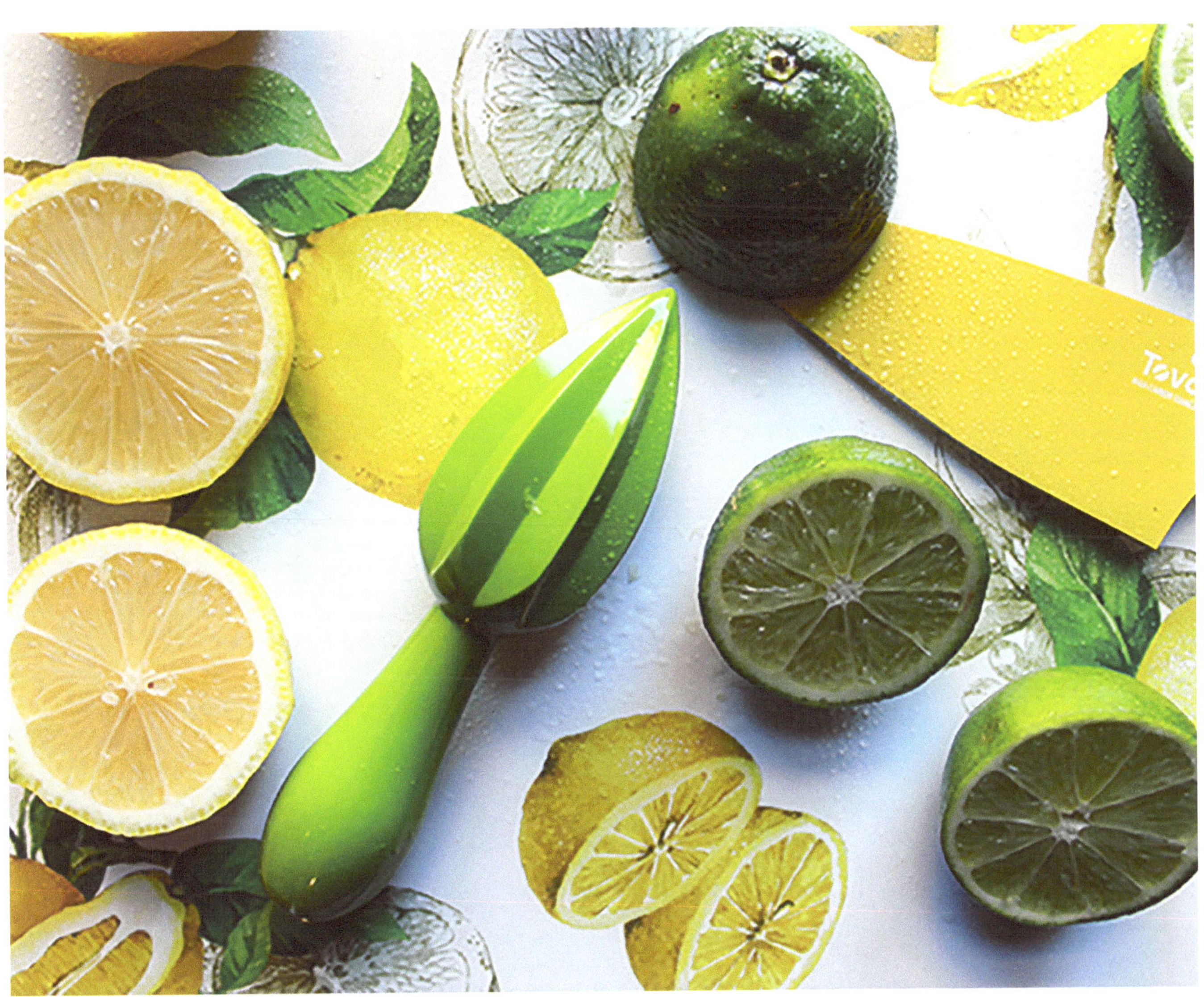

EGGS

CHEF DI'S TIPS

I am wild about eggs! I just love them for their taste and tremendous health benefits. Breakfast. Lunch. Dinner. They are fabulous anytime! I recently heard a Bon Appetit podcast with Editor in Chief, Adam Rappaport where he interviewed actor, Jeff Goldblum about his own love affair with eggs. In this particular episode, Jeff graciously shared his favorite way to cook eggs. He called it, "Scrambled and Rustic." Basically, you crack two large eggs into a frying pan on medium heat and gently drag your spatula back and forth through the middle of them. As the eggs combine with the heat, the whites cook with the whites and the yolks cook with the yolks. When you finish, you have a delightful combination of velvety whites and creamy yolks harmoniously mingled together. The result is pure heaven! Truly divine! It is now one of my new favorite ways to cook eggs.

My niece, Olivia, shared her favorite egg dish with me, and it's delicious. She preheats her oven to 425°F, cuts an avocado in half, removes the pit, and cracks an egg into the hole then she bakes it for 15-20 minutes. This recipe highlights the creaminess in both ingredients and is simply marvelous. I like to add greens to all my eggs to give them some contrast, extra health benefits, and extra love.

I have three rules when preparing my eggs: (1) never overcook them, (2) season them with turmeric, salt, pepper, herbs, hemp and chia seeds, and (3) always add at least one handful of greens in with every egg dish whether it be spinach, winter purslane, baby kale, dandelion greens, micro shungika, scallion greens, or baby white cabbage. The list could go on and on. The great thing about so many of these particular leafy greens is that I did not have to cook them. I place them on my plate, put the warm cooked eggs on top, and enjoy the blend of delicious and flavorful ingredients.

TANYA'S HEALTH BENEFITS

√ Eggs are an excellent source of choline - a neurotransmitter vital for memory, mood, and muscle control as well as vitamins A and D.

√ Choose organic and pasture-raised eggs for the most nutritional value.

√ Look for yolks that are firmer and higher when the egg is cracked (rather than low and flat) and those that are a deeper yellow color. The height signals the egg is fresh, while the color of the yolk indicates the variety of the chicken's diet. A deeper yellow yolk suggests the chicken had access to a wider variety of feed in their diet, which translates to more nutrition in the egg.

√ "Cage-free" may likely be a better choice for eggs. Cage-free eggs are from chickens who have more space to lay their eggs than caged chickens do. If you are greatly concerned about the diet and condition of your chickens, you may need to dig deeper to find out where they lived and what the chickens were fed in order to know about the nutritional value.

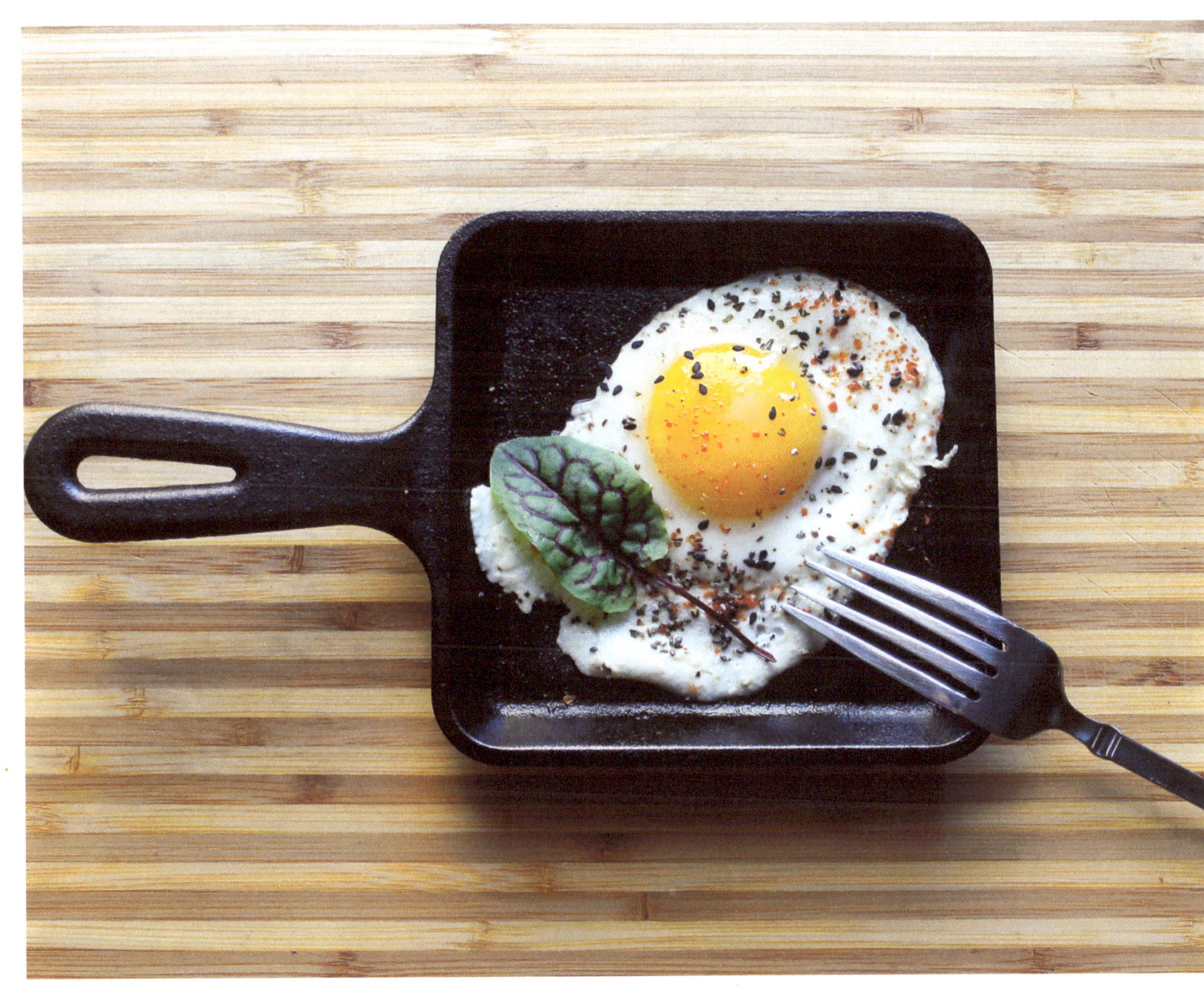

CARROTS

CHEF DI'S TIPS

Full disclosure: I used to snack on those crunchy little baby carrots you find at most supermarkets until I got diagnosed with diabetes. During my research, I discovered my favorite little vegetable was not so good for me. Although quite tasty and not as sweet as fruit, carrots are higher in sugar and carbohydrates than many of my other go-to vegetables. But I do love carrots, so I decided to continue to eat them in moderation. Strolling around the Farmer's Market for carrots is such a fun experience and opened up a whole new world of color and flavor possibilities! These classic organic carrots have a sharper taste and come in a wide array of bright colors, including red, orange, yellow, white, and even purple. When I make my salads now, less is more, so I only toss in a few pretty slices or slivers to add some color and texture. Sometimes I just take the peeler and shred.

Roasted carrots are full of flavor and add a beautiful touch to the canvas of your plate. Here is one of my favorite ways to cook them. Slice the carrot on a diagonal and toss in a bowl with extra virgin olive oil, salt, a dash of curry and a sprinkle of smoky cum-in. Just after you remove them from the oven, scatter a few chopped mint leaves and chives over the top, and you will have a side dish masterpiece a few curly ribbons over the top and mix them in with the other salad goodies.

TANYA'S HEALTH BENEFITS

√ Excellent source of vitamin A - 1 cup of raw carrots provides 428% of your daily value of vitamin A.

√ The antioxidant lutein, a precursor to vitamin A, is found in carrots and helps protect the eye from age-related macular degeneration (AMD), cataracts, and perhaps even diabetes-related damage to the retina.

√ Consume only 1/4 cup of carrots per day to lower your risk of cardiovascular dis-ease.

√ Carrots are a great source of carotenoids, another precursor to vitamin A. However, because this is fat-soluble (stored in your body fat), be wary of eating too many carrots. Not only is the sugar content too high for a diabetic, but you may also start to appear slightly orange. Don't worry, though, this is completely harmless. If you reduce your intake of carrots, you should go back to your normal color within weeks. Fun side note: pumpkins can do this too!

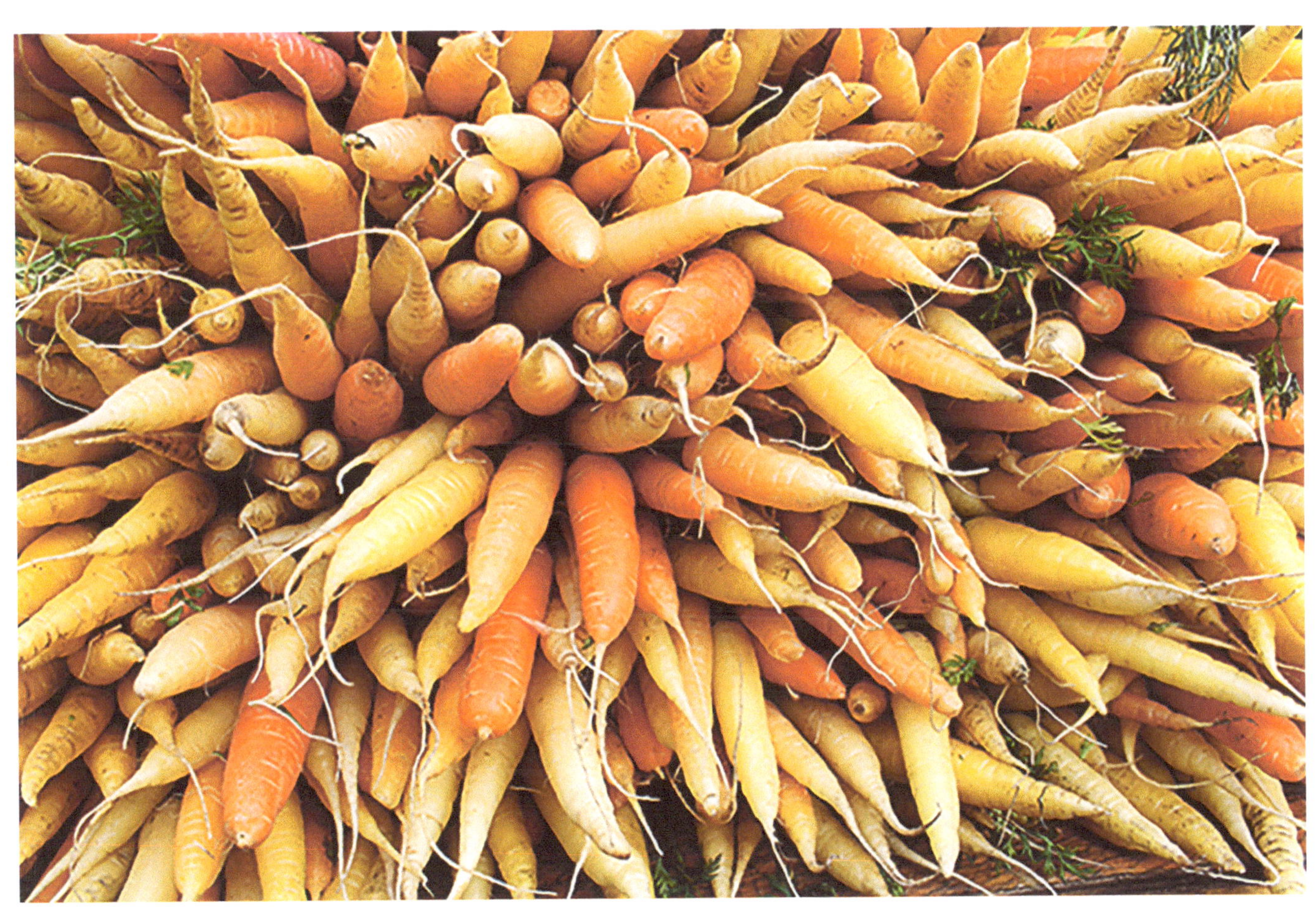

PERSIMMONS

CHEF DI'S TIPS

This wild and wonderful fruit is another new favorite discovery of mine. I would always walk past persimmons at the store and fruit stands and think, "That fruit is not for me. It's too mysterious or too complicated." Ha! How wrong I was! I discovered persimmons are known as "The Fruit of The Gods." These beautiful fruits have a warm orange or yellow hue and a delightfully rich, honey-like sweetness when ripe. The best thing about persimmons is they are one of the healthiest fruits a person can eat. So, as a diabetic who now has to select fruit very carefully, this new information was music to my ears.

The great thing about persimmons is you can eat them hard or slightly soft and ripe. They are great both ways. I love to slice them up and snack on them when I get a craving for something sweet and healthy. My beloved hubby, Billy, loves to blend them up and make juice. You can use persimmons in salads, smoothies, soups, and even as an alternative sweet topping for oatmeal or toast. Persimmons are a wonderful and welcome addition to the fall and winter seasons. They are available around October and carry through to February when most fruits are not accessible! There are so many health benefits to these lovelies, but I will leave that to Tanya to share with us.

TANYA'S HEALTH BENEFITS

√ Choose persimmons with deep red undertones as this means they are ripe and will have the most flavor.
√ One fruit (about 2.5 inches) is 118 calories and 6 grams of fiber. That's almost 25% of the recommended 25 grams of fiber for women per day!
√ That same portion provides 55% of your daily value of vitamin A.
√ Very easy to eat, just slice or eat whole like an apple.
√ Originated in China but brought to the United States in the 1800s.

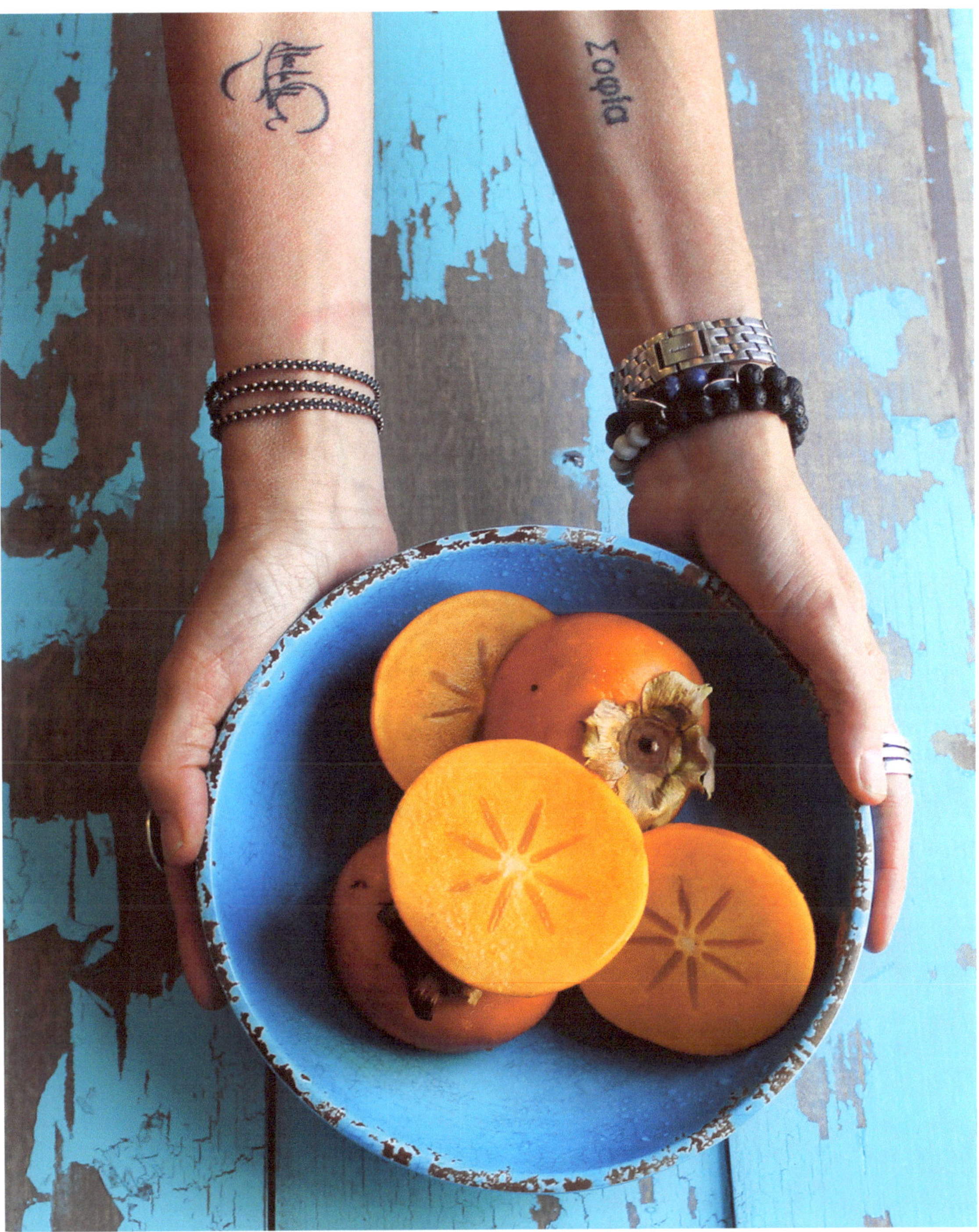
Σοφια

TATSOI

CHEF DI'S TIP

These beautiful leaves have a sweet, pleasant flavor like bok choi or mustard greens but are not as intense. When making a salad, I place them in my friend Margaret Braun's stunning bowl, as seen here, which is an art piece in and of itself.

When I cook tatsoi leaves, I lightly steam or sauté them gently with a clove or two of minced garlic and a small finely chopped shallot. Tatsoi pairs well with everything, but I would lean more towards serving with a fish or chicken dish.

TANYA'S HEALTH BENEFITS

√ Tatsoi is high in vitamins A, C, and K.
√ It is an excellent source of the mineral calcium, potassium, and iron.
√ Another member of the mustard family.

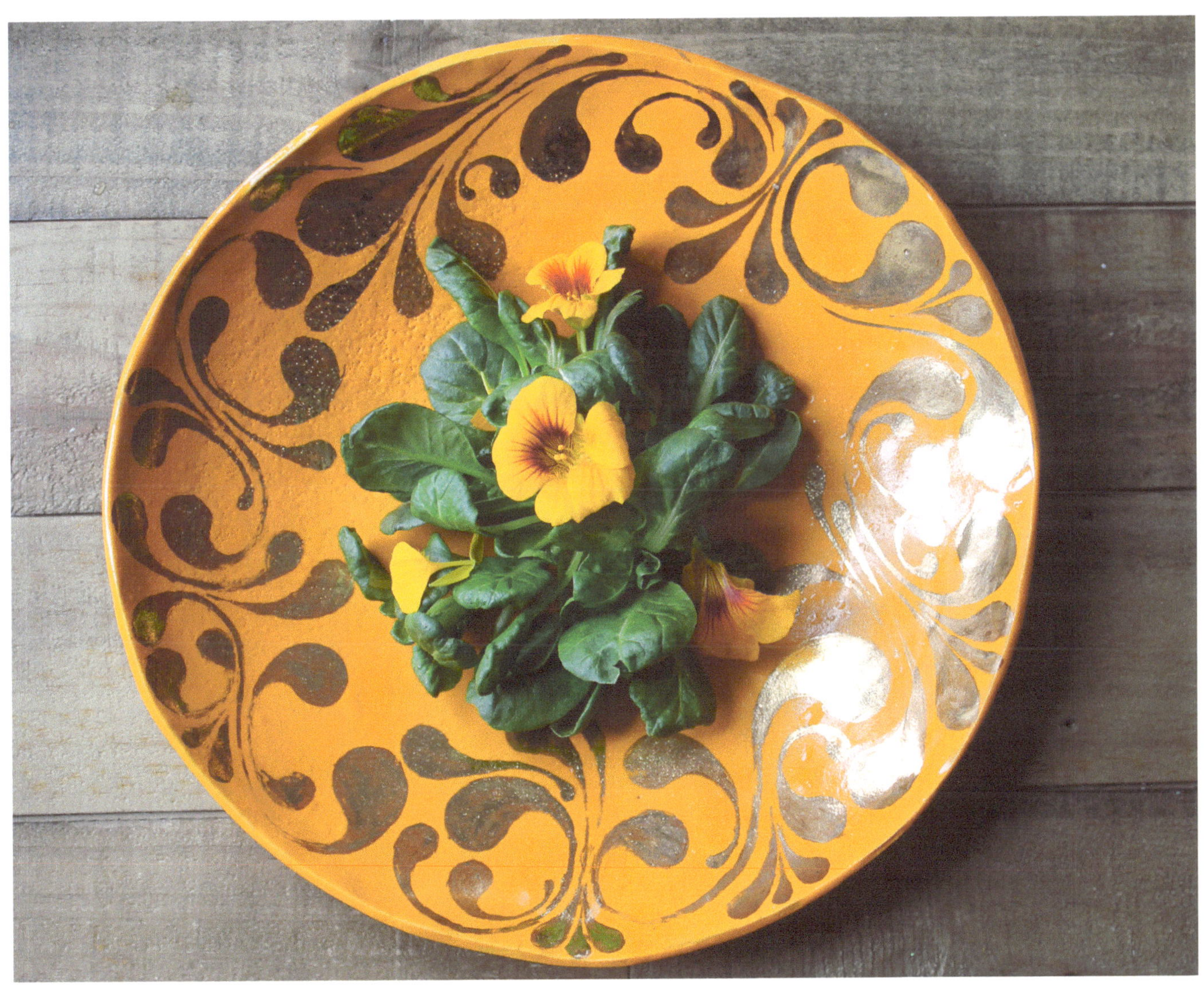

MUSHROOMS

CHEF DI'S TIP

When I was a little girl, I hated mushrooms! 100% truth. Growing up in Europe, whenever my mom would serve them to us, I would always drop the slimy little pieces under the table and feed them to my black Labrador, Charlie. I am not sure if it was the texture or the flavor, but they were so disgusting to me. Even the thought of a mushroom made me shudder. I have to laugh at myself because I crave them all the time now. It's amazing what happens to a person's palate when they become an adult and a chef. I remember in the late 1980s, I went foraging for mushrooms with Chef Tom Valenti and a few other fellow chefs on a tour led by Aux delicies Des Bois in the woods of upstate New York. Believe me, once you pick mushrooms like that from the ground and cook them, your life changes. At least mine did.

I am continually perusing the Farmer's Market seeking out the best selection of these spongy round-top fungi from the finest farmers on the East Coast. For those who are curious, my favorite mushroom farmers so far are Bulich Farms, Gail's Farms, Blue Oyster Cultivation, John D. Madura Farms, and Gajeski Produce.

My suggestion for preparing your mushrooms is—the simpler, the better. Mushrooms that grow in thick nutrient-rich soils are so flavorful, they don't need a lot of seasoning. They can be prepared just as they are. But, if you want to compliment the dish with a little bit of added flavor, I suggest a light sauté or roast with a touch of toasted garlic and a hint of minced shallots. Done and done. Perhaps for presentation, and a splash of color you can add a bit of chive, Thai basil, or even tarragon to finish. But the essence is always the actual mushroom.

Remember my little yellow friend, the lemon? To really spike the natural flavor of a mushroom and give it a little zing, I sprinkle a little bit of lemon zest over the top. I serve mushrooms alongside hot dishes like juicy lamb chops, succulent roasted whole chicken, or even a light, flaky lemon sole. Sometimes, I serve them on a huge platter for "Veggie Night" or toss them with baby greens and a touch of lavender goat cheese, sliced celery, and radishes. Mushrooms are super flexible and do not discriminate. They go with everything, and they make your tummy oh so very happy!

TANYA'S HEALTH BENEFITS

√ The only vegetable source of vitamin D.
√ Choose gray and yellow oyster, shiitake, and maitake mushrooms for the highest boost of antioxidants.
√ One large oyster mushroom has only 63 calories but nearly 5 grams of protein.
√ One large oyster mushroom also contains 25% of the daily value of iron for men and 11% of the daily value of iron for women!
√ Maitake mushrooms work as an adaptogen in the body - a substance that helps fight a variety of stressors as well as boost your immunity.
√ Crimini mushrooms are a great source of copper (essential for healthy red blood cells and iron absorption) and selenium (plays a role in preventing cell damage). In animal studies, shiitake mushrooms have been shown to contain lentinan, a component that may help prevent cancer.
√ Portobello mushrooms are a source of potassium which is excellent for lowering blood pressure. They also contain zinc, which can be helpful for wound healing.
√ Trumpet mushrooms are part of the oyster mushroom family and one of the few mushrooms of which you can eat the stem.

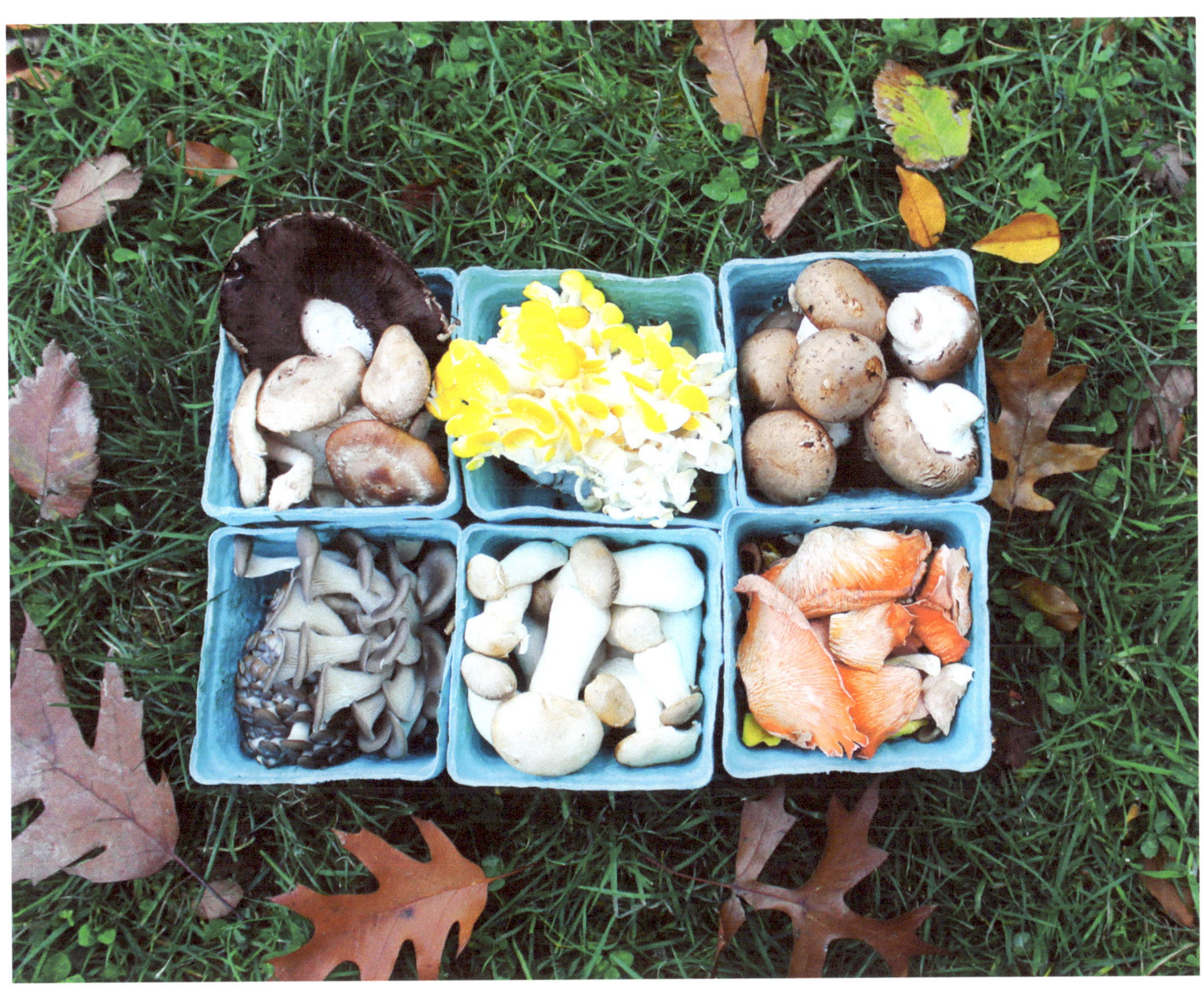

CUCUMBERS

CHEF DI'S TIP

Cucumbers are my go-to snack. I always have them in plastic baggies when I am out and about. This refreshing juicy vegetable goes into every one of my salads. I also like to put them in the infused water I make during the spring and summertime. It tastes so fresh and inviting. Another super easy tip is to use cucumbers as a delicious snack with hummus or to compliment a picnic or brunch. Peel the thick green skin from the lush flesh and slice it into circles, then add a splash of extra virgin olive oil, salt, pepper, a sprinkle of sesame seeds, and freshly chopped basil and mint. Voila!

You can jazz them up and give them a buttery twist by adding a chunky slice of avocado. Or even better, picture yourself on a warm summer day sitting on the veranda of a Mediterranean coast restaurant crunching down on the traditional mix of cucumbers, tomatoes, onions, feta cheese, and tangy Greek olives—all seasoned with delicious olive oil, lime juice, and zest, and kissed with the perfect hint of oregano. Where would a Greek salad be without the cucumbers?

The cucumbers in the photo are called sanditas (little watermelon or little mouse melon). These tiny delights are super crunchy and have a vibrant lemony flavor! I found a gold mine of them during one of my Farmer's Market trips at the Windfall Farms booth, and they are the best! These luscious minis are not around until around July, but so worth the wait.

TANYA'S HEALTH BENEFITS

√ Low-calorie - only 16 calories per cup. Excellent diuretic - helps eliminate water retention and bloating.
√ Excellent source of vitamin K - helps with blood clotting.

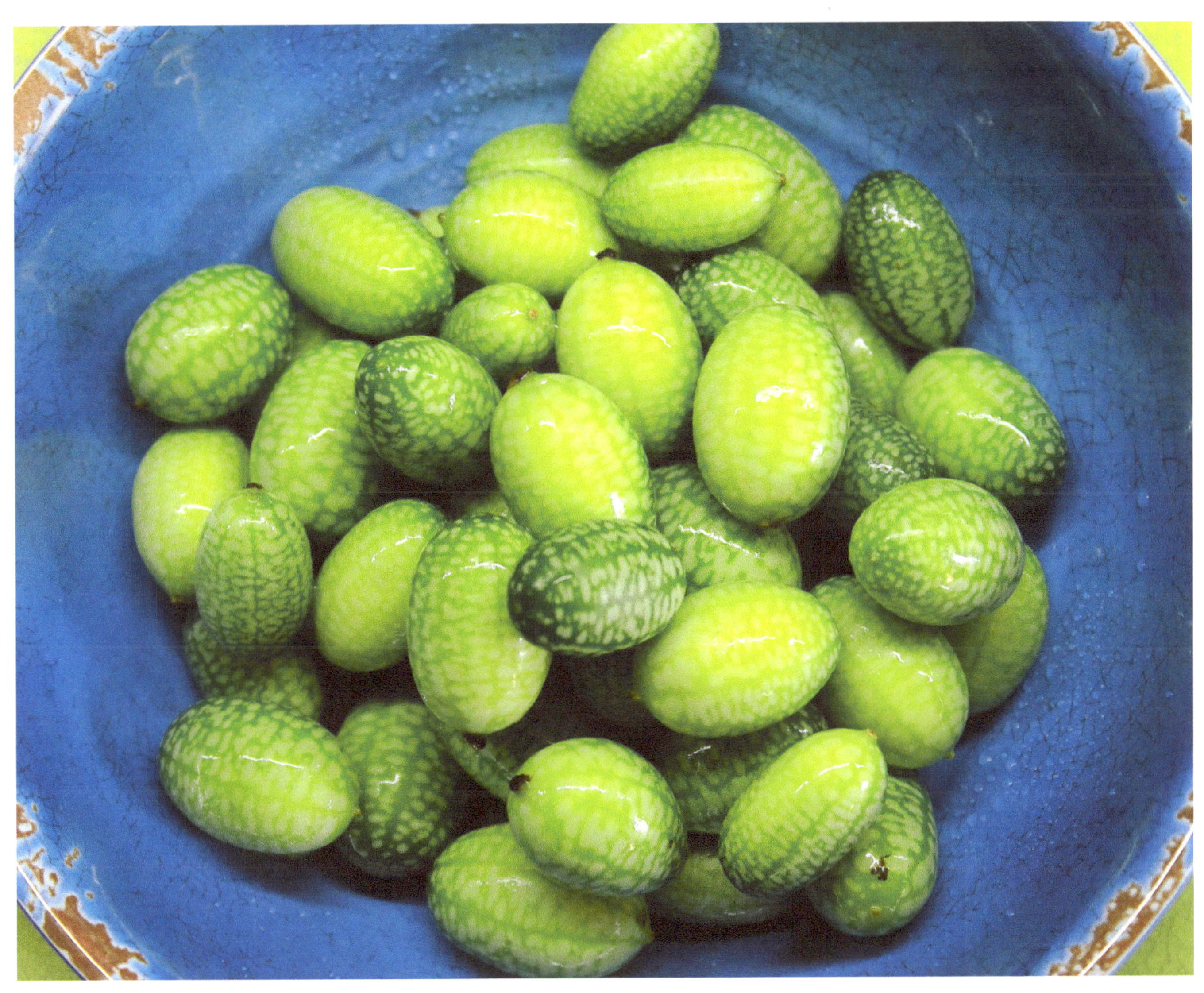

SARDINES

CHEF DI'S TIP

This picture is extra special for me. These mouth-watering sardines are simply divine. In Southern Spain, where my Papa and Pam live, there is a quaint coast side restaurant called Las Flores. Every time I visit, I devour at least two plates of these delicious briny sardines. The chefs in this delightful restaurant pull these small fish right out of the water and throw them onto a smoking grill where they are simply basted with olive oil and lemon. That's honestly all they need!

I have yet to find any of my favorite restaurants in New York City who serve sardines, but I am still looking. Sardines do not need much pampering and can be eaten on their own just like the picture shows or you can break them up and place the pieces on top of beautiful greens with some salty capers and sweet grilled peaches. They can even be tossed into a bowl of crisp cucumbers and ripe tomatoes. Personally, I think when they are served on their own, it honors them the way they deserve to be honored.

Now I know that people may think sardines only come in a can, they taste extremely fishy and smell really bad. But trust me, if you are open and give them a chance, you might just be surprised. I promise.

TANYA'S HEALTH BENEFITS

√ A fantastic source of vitamin B12 - 137% of your daily value in only one can.
√ One can of sardines contains 35% of your daily value of calcium - more than a glass of milk or cup of yogurt.
√ Great source of heart-healthy omega-3 fatty acids - the type of fat known to reduce inflammation in the body and lower triglyceride levels.
√ Due to their small size, sardines are incredibly low in mercury compared to other healthy fatty fish like tuna and salmon.

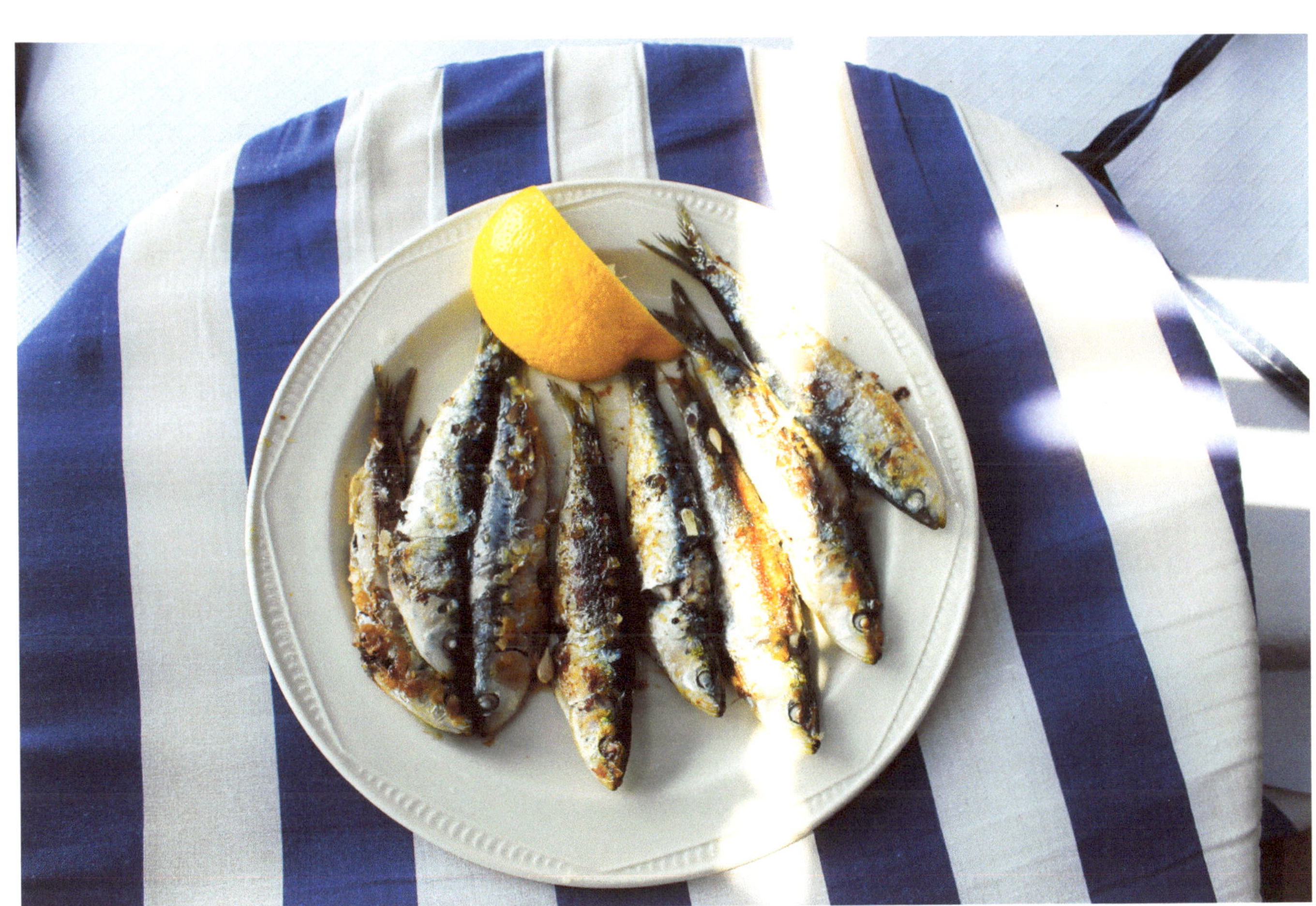

TURNIPS

CHEF DI'S TIP

Turnips. The plain and simple truth is I never really loved them. That is until I found these little white gems at the Farmer's Market. Having them sourced organically from the local farmers here in on the East Coast makes a world of difference in the flavor, and it is astounding. These baby turnips called Hakurai Japanese turnips are from Windfall Farms, and they taste like candy. As a diabetic who misses her sweets, these are a great substitute. Cupcakes or turnips? Drumroll…and the winner for me, is turnips.

Preparing them as a snack or side dish is incredibly easy. Drizzle with some extra virgin olive oil, then sprinkle with salt, cracked black pepper, chopped dried herbs, and a dash of crushed red pepper flakes. Toss them in a bowl, put them in the oven at 350°F, and roast until done. While baking, the edges will turn a little brown, and start to caramelize. That is the sweetness coming out. Oh, so good.
P.S. Turnips come with an added gift—the turnip greens. I recommend chopping them off and steaming or sautéing them separately for just a few seconds.

TANYA'S HEALTH BENEFITS

√ Eat both the root and the turnip greens for the most nutrition.
√ 1 cup of raw greens provides 173% of your daily value of vitamin K - vital for proper blood clotting.
√ 1 cup of raw greens provides 10% of your daily value of calcium.
√ Part of the cruciferous vegetable family - like broccoli and kale, turnips and turnip greens share many of the same fantastic health benefits.
√ Try grated turnips in place of cabbage for a new twist on coleslaw.

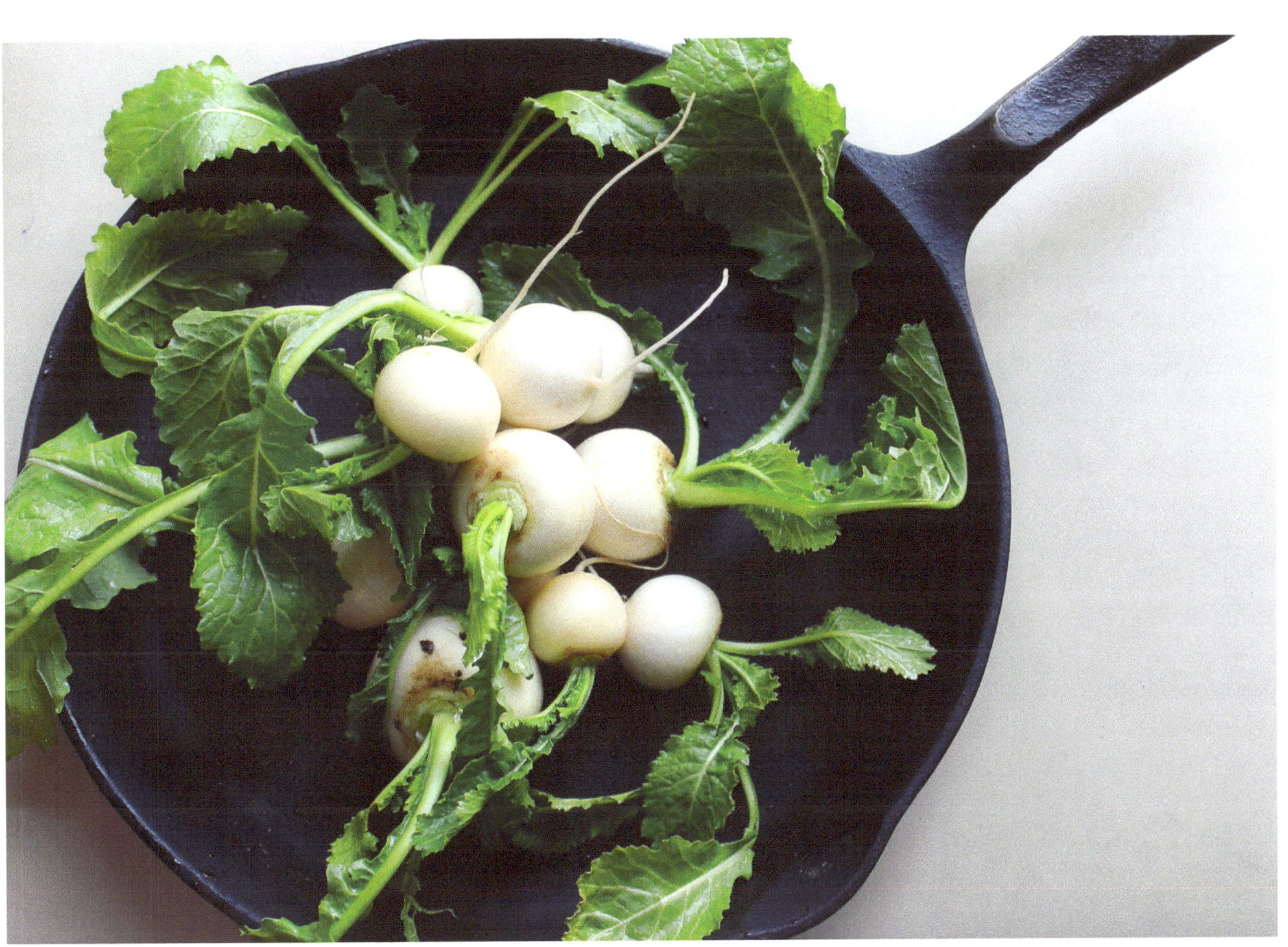

HEMP & CHIA

CHEF DI'S TIP

These two earthy ingredients are entirely new to me, and I just love them both! When I found out how many health benefits were squeezed into these tiny little seeds, it made me want to use and enjoy them that much more. I'll admit, it is the smooth, pleasant flavor I crave so much. Especially the hemp seeds. The nutty taste compliments many of my dishes from yogurts to salads to any entrée. And of course, you will find them in my snack bag too.

TANYA'S HEALTH BENEFITS

√ Chia seeds are a great source of protein and omega-3 fatty acids.
√ Hemp hearts are easy to digest as well as high in heart-healthy unsaturated fats, fiber, protein, iron, and potassium.
√ Hemp hearts (the hulled version of hemp seeds) are a soft textured and mild tasting choice within the nut and seed family.
√ Absorb up to ten times their weight in water.
√ My favorite way to eat them is as chia pudding. Mix 1-2 tablespoons with unsweetened almond milk, mix well and refrigerate overnight. In the morning you'll have a delicious, filling, high-fiber pudding to top with either fresh berries or chopped apple and cinnamon. Yummy and so good for you!

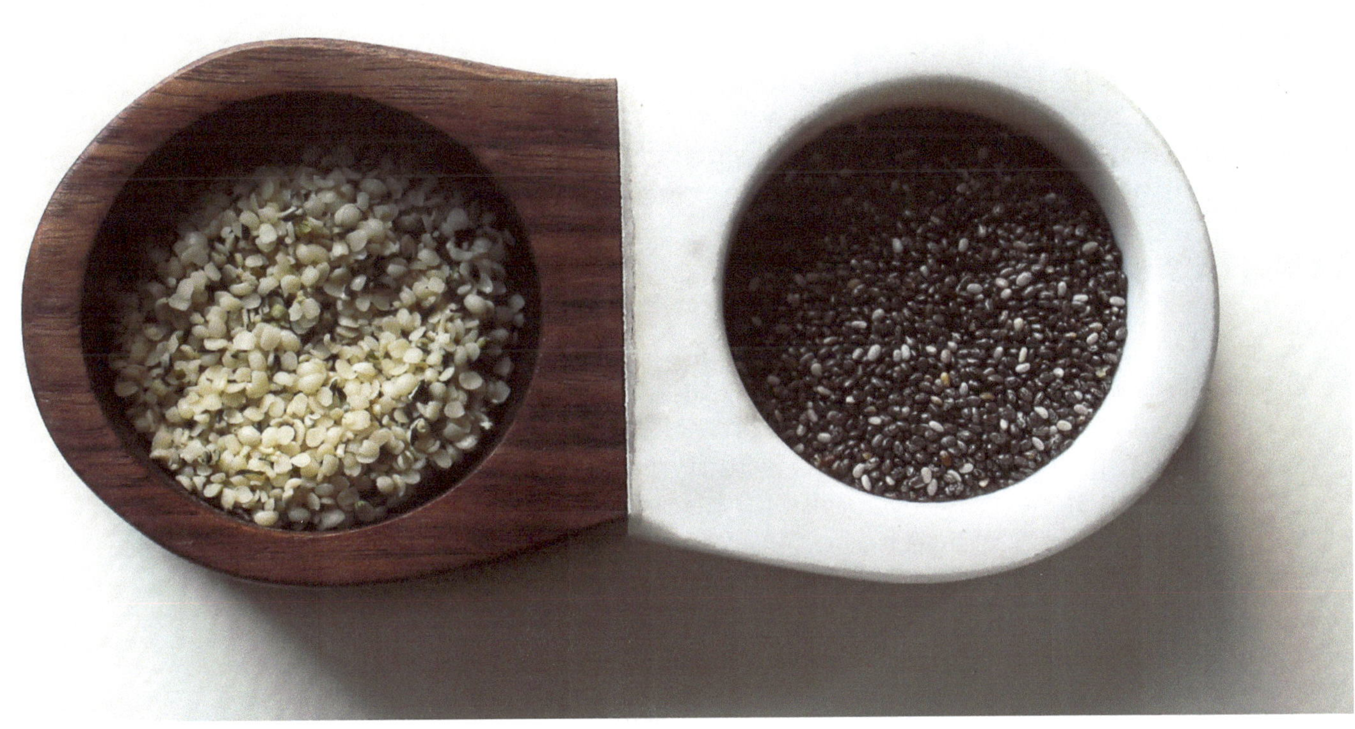

RED CABBAGE

CHEF DI'S TIP

Red cabbage is another new favorite vegetable of mine. I never really spent much time eating it, but now that I gave it a chance, I have it in my fridge all the time. I shred it and add it to every one of my salad mixes. I even keep it raw in my snack bag, mainly for the pleasure of the texture. Red cabbage is a perfect peppery yet sweet addition to a savory roast chicken or salty roast pork dish. I usually shred it into long red ribbons and place it around the roasts when they are close to finishing. Sometimes I cook it down with a seasoned broth and freshly chopped herbs to make a savory side dish. This not only adds beautiful vibrant color to your plate but also compliments both meat and vegetable dishes.

TANYA'S HEALTH BENEFITS

√ High in a flavonoid called anthocyanin - antioxidants that may boost brain health and prevent cancer. Excellent source of vitamin A, C, fiber, and iron.
√ 1 cup of raw red cabbage also provides 85% of your daily value of vitamin C.
√ Consumption of red cabbage is known to lower LDL cholesterol, a type of harmful cholesterol that increases your risk for heart disease.
√ 1 cup of raw cabbage has only 27 calories. Combined with its fiber content, it keeps you feeling full and satisfied using minimal calories

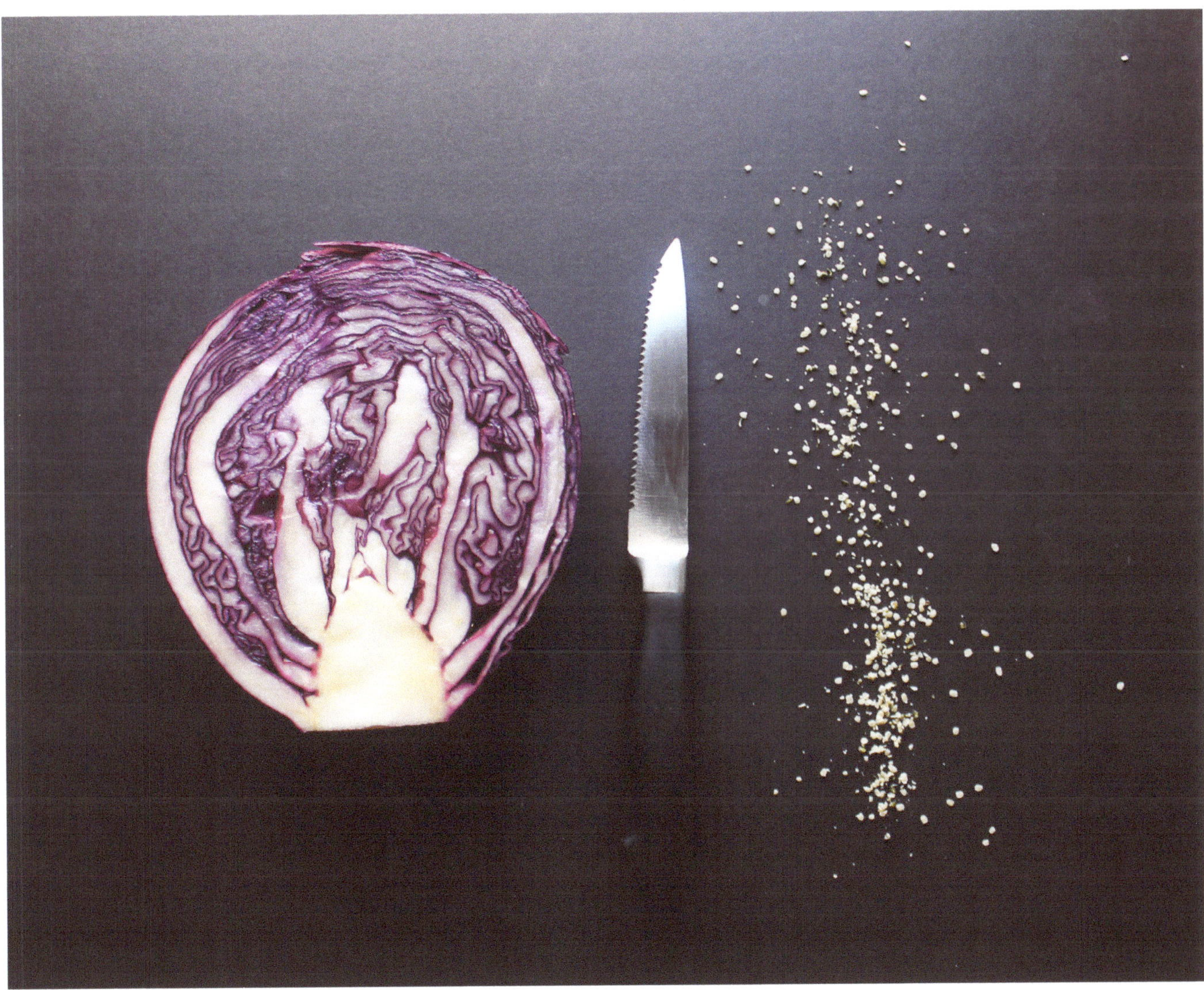

RADISHES

CHEF DI'S TIP

I never used to be a big fan of radishes. I found their sharp taste too strong for my liking. Then I got brave and started exploring the radishes at my local Farmer's Market. Once I finally took a chance on these little pearls, my entire outlook changed. From watermelon radishes to purple, green, black, and daikon—the varieties and wide-range of exciting colors are endless! Most importantly, when you get them fresh from the soil, the flavor is one-hundred times better than those found in any local supermarket. Like turnips, there is a smooth sweetness to them, and I can enjoy them like candy. Yet another substitute for my sweet tooth!

During the summer months, I find the smaller radishes tend to have a juicy tenderness to them. They are also visually stunning and make the perfect eye-catching artistic compliment to any presentation. From a photographer's point of view, they create the winning shot. I usually slice my radishes paper thin or chop them into small rectangular boxes then use them as a garnish on my salads. I even garnish my entrée dishes. And of course, they are a regular in my snack bag. One more wonderful added bonus—they are available year-round. So when you venture out on your weekly walk through the local Farmer's Market, try a radish. I think you will thank me.

TANYA'S HEALTH BENEFITS

√ Part of the cruciferous vegetable family - cruciferous vegetables are known for the prevention of cancer by inhibiting enzymes that activate carcinogens and turn on tumor suppressor genes.
√ Helpful for lowering LDL cholesterol - a type of cholesterol that raises heart disease risk.
√ Nearly 30% of your daily value of vitamin C.
√ 1 cup of radishes has only 20 calories.
√ Great source of fiber - 2 grams in one cup of slices

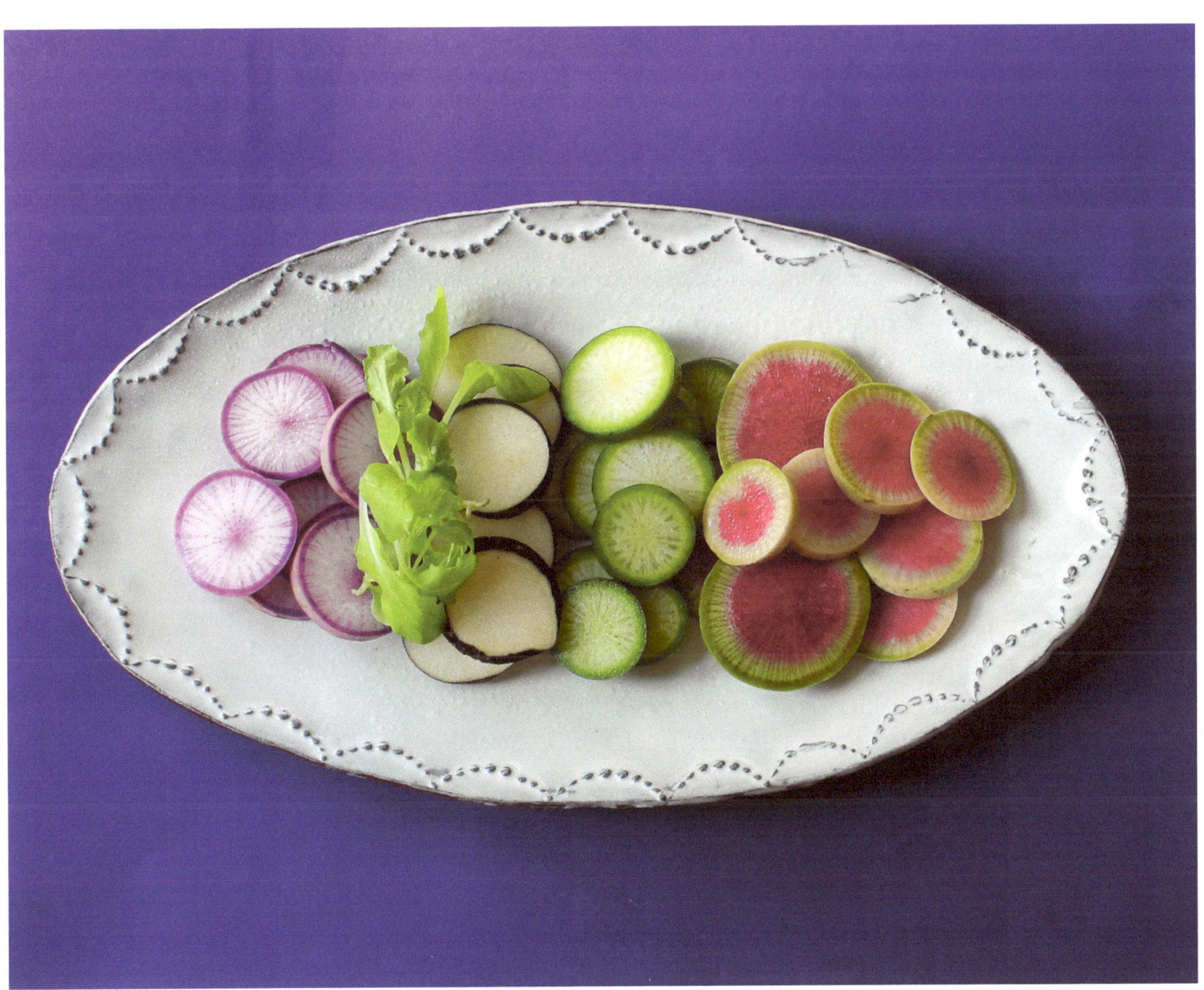

POMEGRANATES

CHEF DI'S TIP

Pomegranates are another new favorite ingredient of mine. I always thought it was too much work to crack open that thick purple skin and dig out those plump little kernels. But after realizing how wonderfully healthy and beneficial they are, I add them to my salads, cashew yogurt, and soups as a garnish. I have even found it brings a sweet and sour note to roast chicken dishes as well as fish dishes. Pomegranate also pairs quite nicely with fennel and leeks.

TANYA'S HEALTH BENEFITS

√ A fantastic source of polyphenols and antioxidants.
√ Heart-healthy source of fiber.
√ High content of vitamin C protects skin from damage.
√ An average pomegranate has up to 600 seeds!

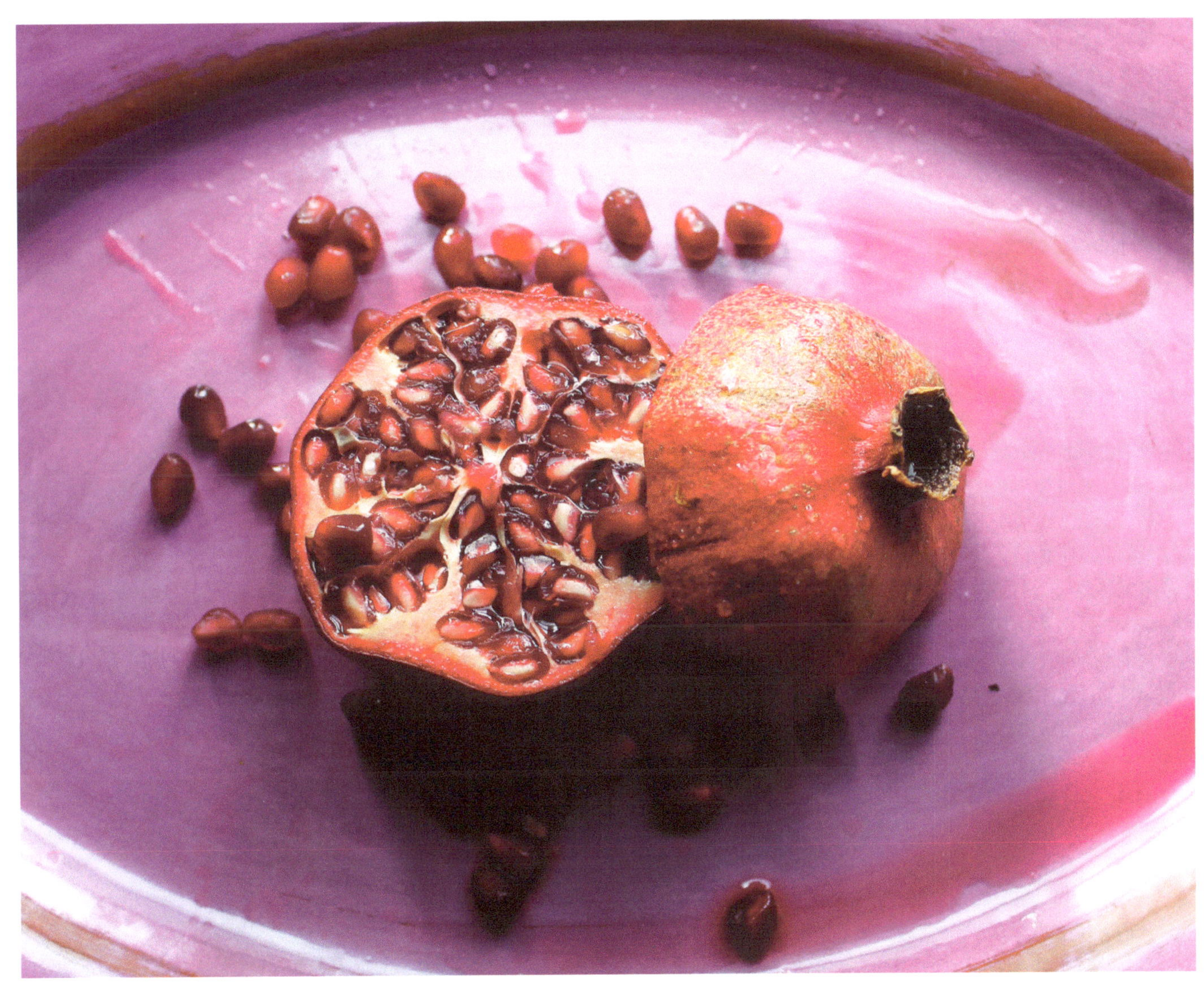

FiGS

CHEF DI'S TIP

Luckily, with the limited list of fruits I can eat, figs are one that I can. I am crazy about figs. I love the flavor, the look, all of it. Figs can be paired with so many beautiful sweet and savory dishes. Its pulpy sweetness gives honey-like undertones and a nice rich flavor. In this pictured dish, I paired the figs with cashew yogurt, and winter purslane leaves from our local farmer, Two Guys from Woodbridge. While I am not a fan of fruit with entrée dishes, I will usually pair figs with roasted lamb chops or grilled salmon.

My favorite memory of eating figs brings me back to Turkey when I was working on my documentary project called, Faces of Tomorrow, right after the devastating earthquake in 1999. In between shoots, when I stopped for breaks, I would return to my tent to find Turkish women cooking on little make-shift stovetops. The men working with them picked fresh figs for me to snack on from the fig tree still standing outside the tent while I waited. Those rich, sweet flavors and tender memories of the generosity of the Turkish people will be in my heart forever.

TANYA'S HEALTH BENEFITS

√ Excellent source of fiber at 1.5 grams per fig.
√ You can use fig puree to replace both the fat and some of the added sugars in baked goods recipes.
√ Figs contain probiotics - the type of fiber that feeds the good bacteria in your digestive system.
√ One fig is an excellent source of potassium and contains 4% of your daily value as well as B vitamins and calcium.
√ Be cautious with dried figs. 100 grams of dried figs contains 48 grams of sugar - more than your entire day's recommended sugar intake.
√ Recent studies are exploring if figs can actually help manage diabetes due to their high antioxidant content.
√ The fig tree flowers are actually inside the fruit!

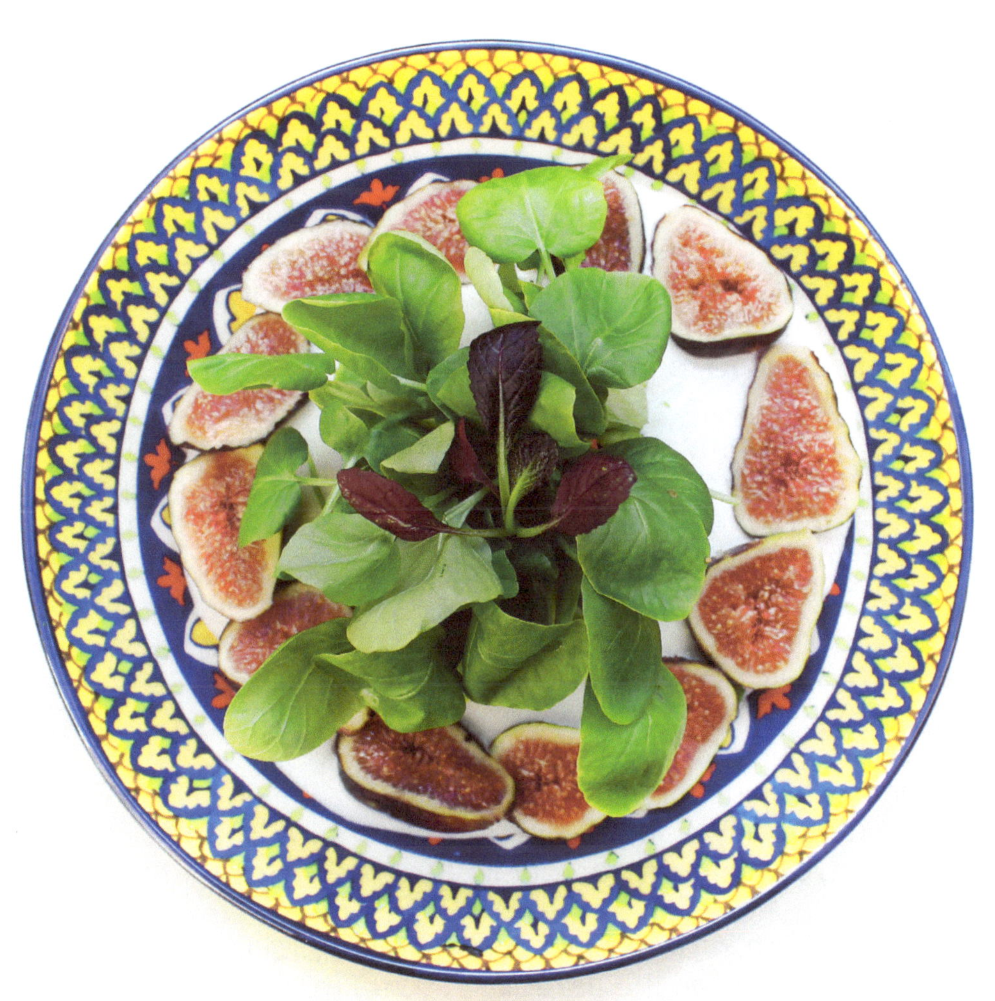

RED SORREL

CHEF DI'S TIP

Sorrel has always been a favorite of mine. I use this leafy herb to add a fun tarty sour note to a variety of vegetable dishes and soups. It is especially good with the roasted leek and garlic dish I serve with grilled salmon or my braised tomato-herbed halibut. The super tangy flavor blends beautifully with the creaminess of fish.

Red sorrel is a new love for me. When I met my new friend Eric, a farmer from Two Guys from Woodbridge, he introduced me to these lovely little red leaves, and I decided to give them a try. They are more delicate than sorrel with a whole lot of flavor. Like sorrel, there is a slight tartness to them, but the tang is milder than regular sorrel. When I use red sorrel, I don't even cook it. I just add it to my cooked dishes, and it wilts beautifully. I also tear pieces of the leaves and add it to my salads. Red Sorrel is pretty in any dish.

TANYA'S HEALTH BENEFITS

√ Helpful to reduce sinus congestion and headaches.
√ Sorrel is high in vitamin A and C.
√ Red sorrel contains phytochemicals and flavonoids, such as quercetin that are potent antioxidants. Quercetin, in particular, may help protect the brain from damage over time.
√ Red sorrel is also high in potassium, a mineral helpful to lower blood pressure.
√ Red sorrel is different than the Jamaican sorrel (hibiscus).
√ Looks like spinach leaves, but sorrel leaves have a sharp tart taste.

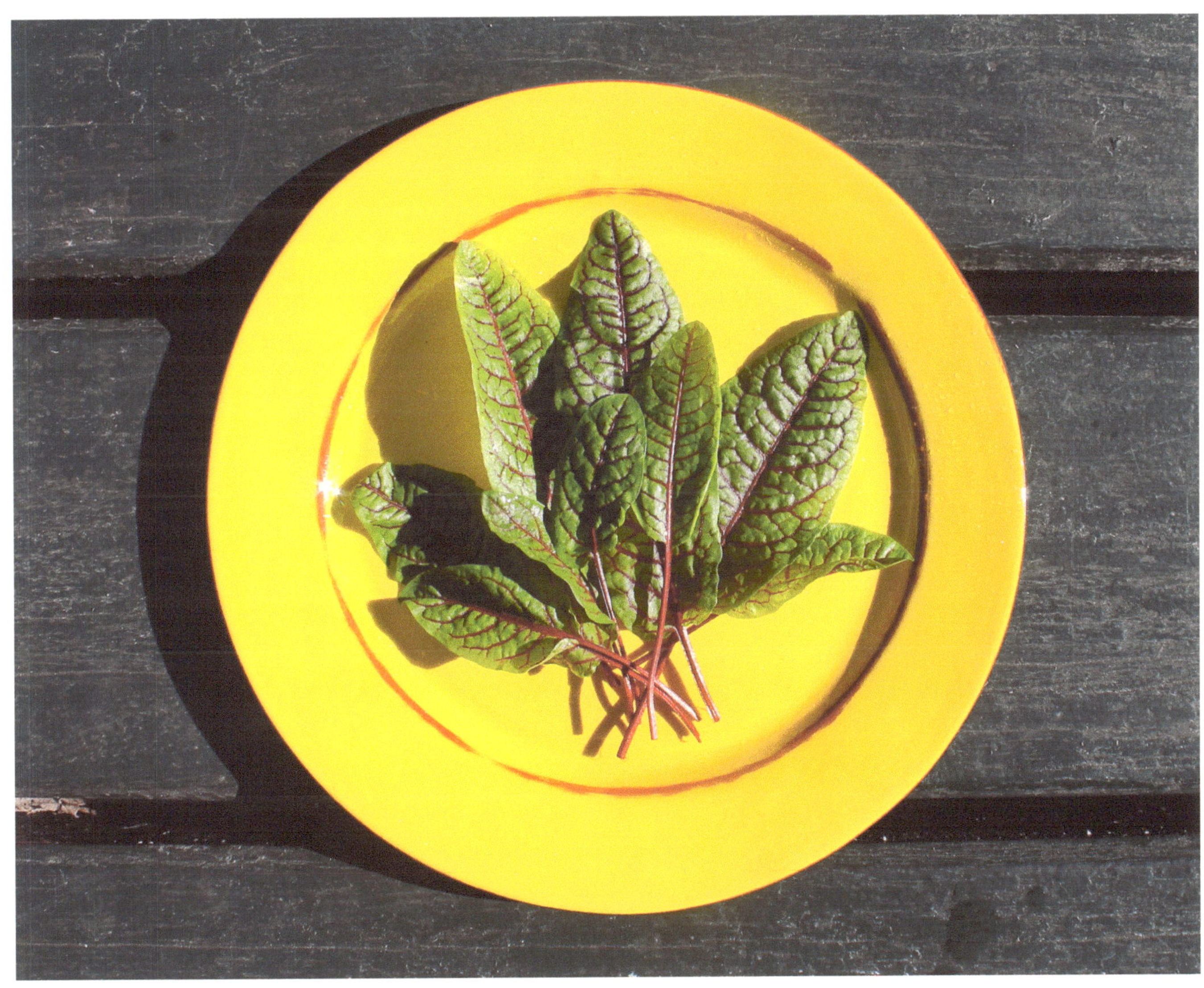

SQUASH BLOSSOMS

CHEF DI'S TIP

I am one of the luckiest girls alive because I was literally born in paradise—Florence, Italy. While we did not live in Italy for long, I feel I am truly 100% Italian. Squash blossoms are one of the Italian people's favorite delicacies. Here in New York City, I look forward to the two or three week window during the summertime when I can find these babies at the Farmer's Market. Oh, I am so happy when they arrive! There are so many things you can do with them. I stuff them with herbed goat cheese, or sausage, or tiny chopped vegetables. Sometimes I lightly fry them or roast them. I have even shredded them into an omelet or a salad. Their flavor and visual beauty are both stunning. Don't be afraid to experiment and have fun with this unexpected little treat. Go for it.

TANYA'S HEALTH BENEFITS

√ Very low in calories but high in vitamin A and C.
√ High in potassium and magnesium – both helpful for keeping your heart rate and blood pressure in a healthy range.
√ Extremely perishable and hard to find in stores. Look for them at your Farmer's Market.
√ Their flavor matches their availability—light and fleeting!
√ If you are allergic to these foods, take care to avoid the blossoms, even with the stamen and pistils removed, it can cause an allergic reaction.

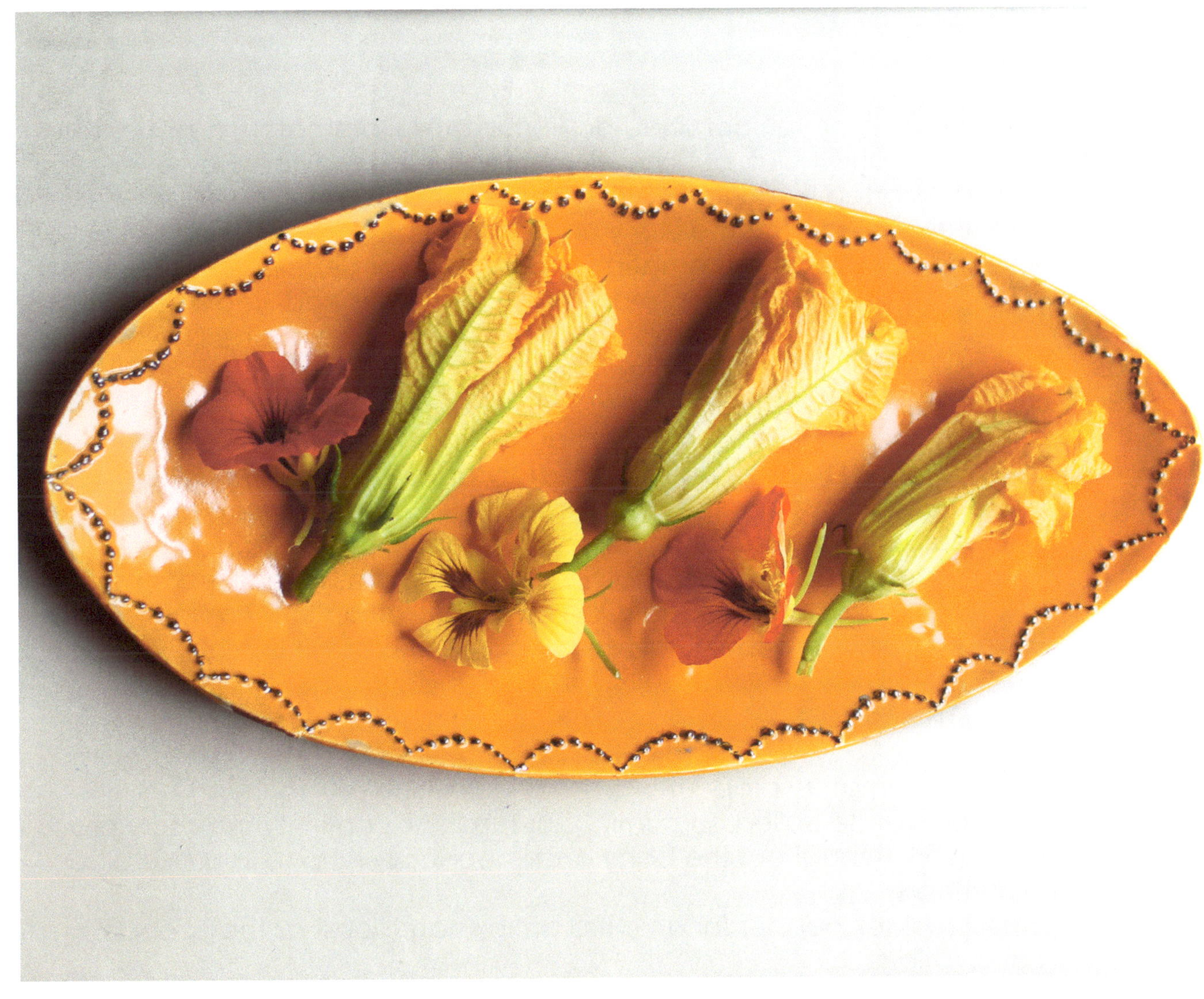

TURMERIC

CHEF DI'S TIP

For years I heard turmeric contained powerful anti-inflammatory qualities and should be added to one's diet, but I never listened to that advice. However, after I got diagnosed, I started learning about cooking with turmeric. The health benefits are absolutely essential for me in my new healing process. Little did I know that I would fall in love with the aromatic flavor of this wonderful spice! I put it on everything from eggs to vegetables to oatmeal and so on. And, you'll never taste anything better than a juicy roast chicken with turmeric butter rubbed all over it! So delicious. Always remember to add black pepper when using it.

If you are really adventurous, it makes a delightful spicy tea. Golden milk is an excellent end to a long day, and its inflammatory properties will help to relieve any fatigue. Take a cup of any kind of milk you choose (I like coconut milk), add 1/2 teaspoon of turmeric, 1/4 teaspoon of cinnamon (optional), some grated fresh ginger, and a pinch of black pepper. It is so soothing and nurturing. When I really need a great night's sleep, this is my go-to tea! One major tip, turmeric does stain, so beware. I own many yellow tea towels!

TANYA'S HEALTH BENEFITS

√ Potent anti-inflammatory properties are particularly helpful for heart health.
√ Contains a substance called curcumin. Curcumin has anti-inflammatory properties that can work throughout the body and specifically help to improve blood cholesterol numbers.
√ Combine with black pepper for an extra antioxidant boost as they cooperate for increased absorption.

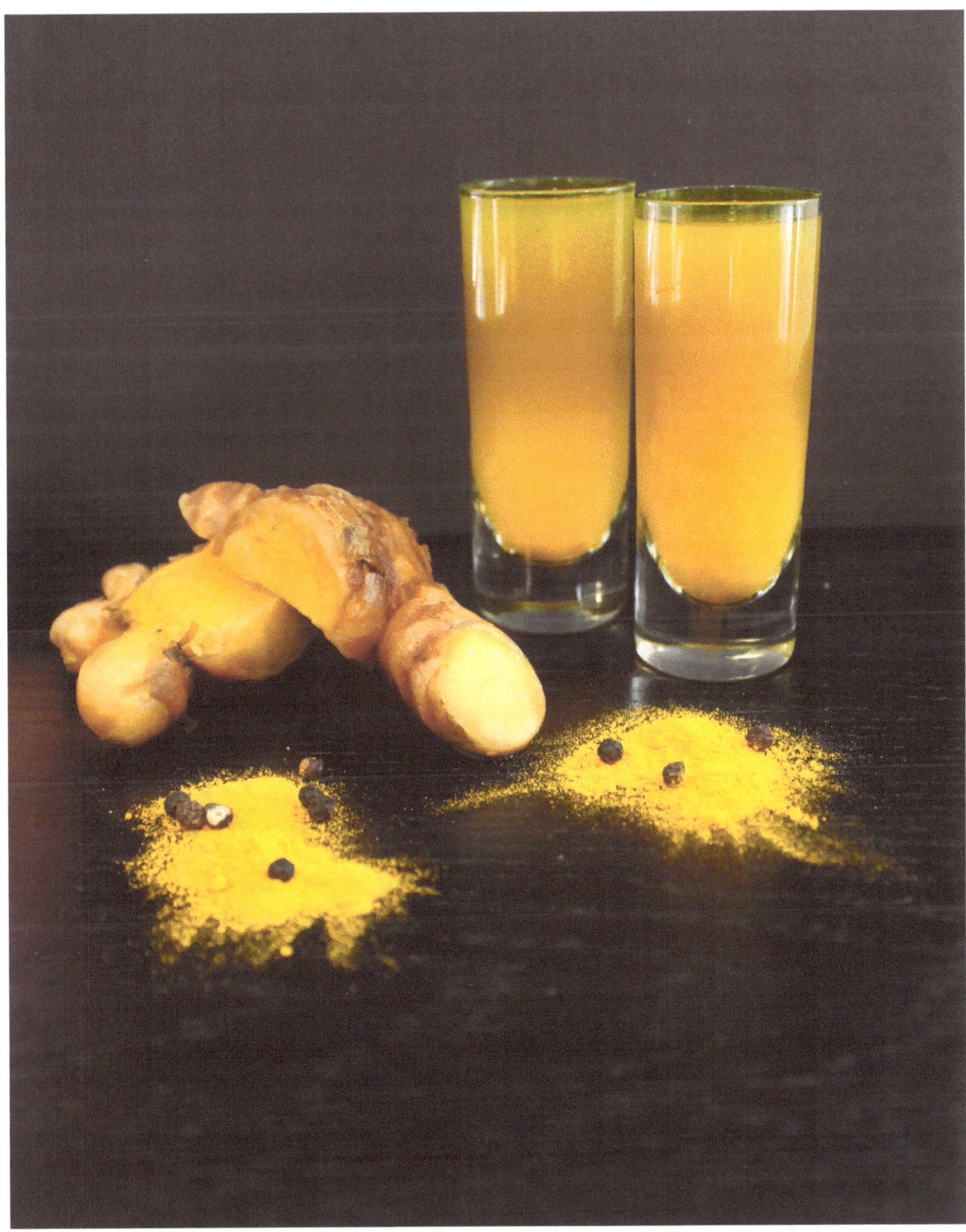

MIXED GREENS

CHEF DI'S TIP

My happy place is looking at a table full of fresh, crisp Farmer's Market greens. I eat greens for all three of my meals, even snacks. One great tip for full flavor is to add herbs to the greens. I just use the fresh herbs I keep on hand, tear them into pieces, and toss them into the salad bowl. I tend to dress the greens very lightly by using a splash of extra virgin olive oil and a squeeze of lemon or lime. Fresh organic greens have so much flavor on their own, they barely need a vinaigrette, but I make a small jar of vinaigrette every week, so I have it if I need it for my salads. This light dressing consists of a dash of wet mustard, a big squeeze of lemon, a drizzle of water, sliced shallots, chopped herbs, and extra virgin olive oil.

If I am eating the greens with a cooked dish, for example, an egg or a dinner entrée, I will most likely not cook the greens. The heat from the food is good enough. But, if the greens are a little tougher and have thicker leaves like mustard greens, dandelion, or even spinach, I will sauté some minced garlic and chopped onions, then add the greens to the hot pan for just under a minute.

TANYA'S HEALTH BENEFITS

√ Baby butter lettuce - 1 cup of lettuce only contains 7 calories and 1 gram of carbohydrates.
√ Baby kale - a great source of vitamin K, vitamin A, vitamin C, fiber, and carotenoids without the toughness and bitterness of adult kale bunches.
√ Spinach - a fantastic source of potassium, spinach can be useful in reducing blood pressure. Spinach is also a fantastic source of iron!
√ Arugula- may offer protection against prostate, breast, cervical, colon, and ovarian cancers by inhibiting cancer cell growth. Also, very high in folate - an incredibly essential nutrient during pregnancy.
√ Kohlrabi - as part of the cruciferous vegetable family, kohlrabi can help lower your blood cholesterol numbers.
√ Mizuna - a member of the mustard family - high in vitamin K which helps with blood clotting. Tatsoi - another member of the mustard family - high in vitamins A, C, and K as well as the minerals calcium, potassium, and iron.
√ Baby Shungiku - also known as crown daisy or chrysanthemum greens - a great source of potassium, antioxidants, fiber, calcium, and iron.
√ Rainbow Swiss Chard - high in nitrates (similar to beets) - may be especially helpful in reducing blood pressure and improving the health of the blood vessel lining known as the endothelium.
√ Purple Leaf Lettuce - excellent source of vitamin A, K, and fiber. Vitamin K is vital for bone health and blood clotting.
√ Snow Pea Shoots - great source of folate - a vitamin absolutely necessary during pregnancy to avoid spina bifida (a dangerous condition for a developing fetus).

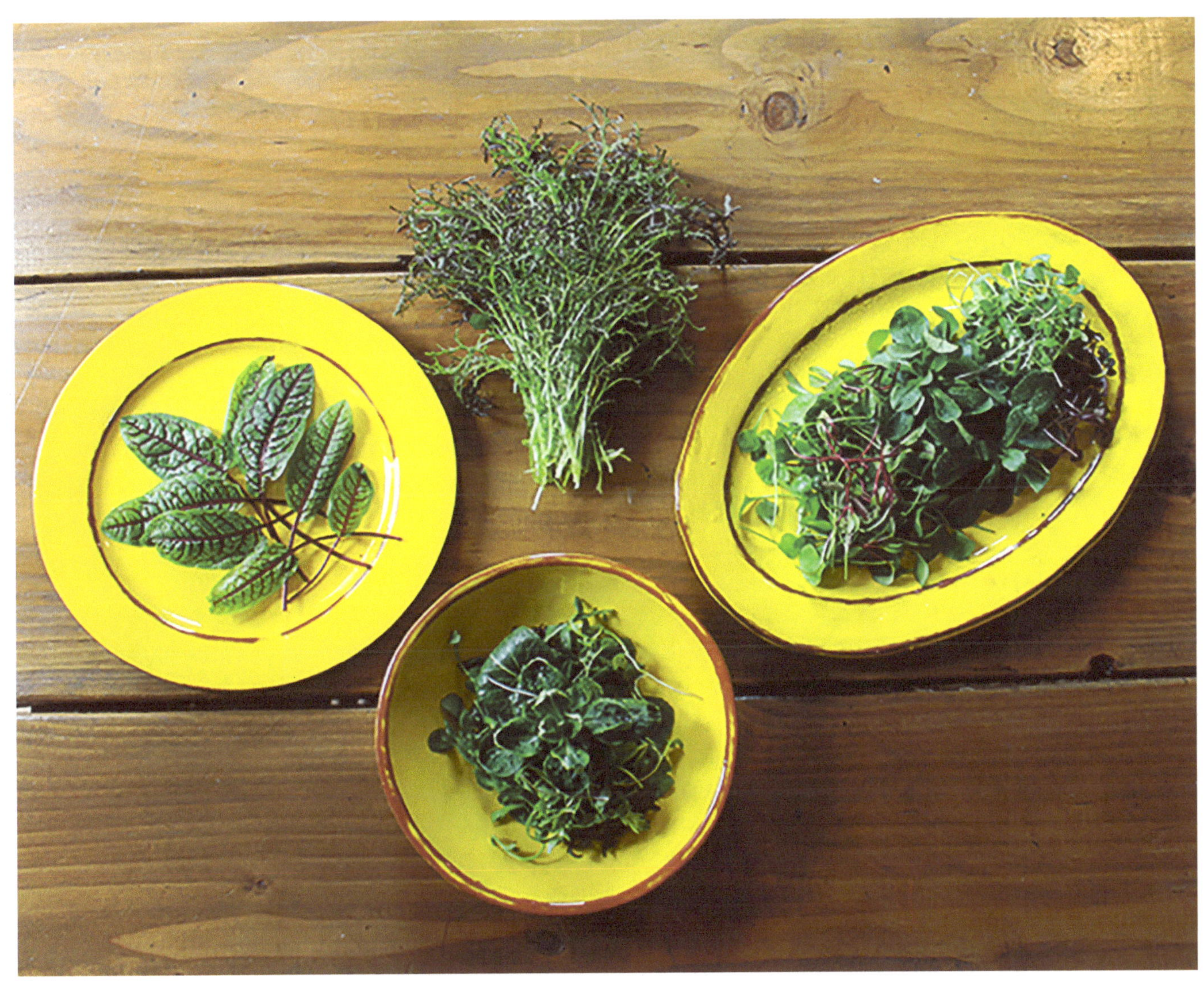

TOMATOES

CHEF DI'S TIP

There is nothing better than a gorgeously ripe, juicy tomato on a hot summer's day. The great thing about tomatoes is they are fabulous to eat on their own. Or, you can slice them and drizzle a little bit of extra virgin olive oil, sprinkle a few pieces of basil leaf, and add a dash of salt and pepper. That's it! I'll admit, I also love to enjoy a platter of roasted tomatoes with a batch of creamy wild mushroom and chive scrambled eggs. I cut the tomatoes in half and lay them on a foil-covered baking sheet, drizzle extra virgin olive oil, herbs de Provence, and a touch of salt and pepper over the top then I roast them in the oven at 350°F for 20 minutes. The smell alone will transform your kitchen into a beautiful countryside garden nestled beneath the hills of Tuscany! I always add tomatoes to the chicken and fish stews I make. The recipes are endless! My only real tip here is to get really good tomatoes, preferably at the local Farmer's Market. If you can't find any there, try to shop around. It's worth the extra search for a good tomato.

TANYA'S HEALTH BENEFITS

√ One cup of cherry tomatoes only has 27 calories, but 32% of your daily value for vitamin C. Excellent source of lycopene - an antioxidant that helps to reduce inflammation and oxidative stress in the body. Common causes of oxidative stress are smoking, pollution, and a processed, Western diet.

√ Lycopene is a red carotenoid pigment that not only lends its red coloring to tomatoes but is also the precursor to carotene or vitamin A in the body.

√ Studies have shown more health benefits come from consuming tomatoes rather than taking lycopene supplements. And there are even more benefits that come from consuming cooked or processed tomatoes rather than just eating raw tomatoes.

√ The bioavailability of lycopene increases further when eaten with dietary fat.

√ Let tomatoes ripen on the counter. They lose their flavor when refrigerated.

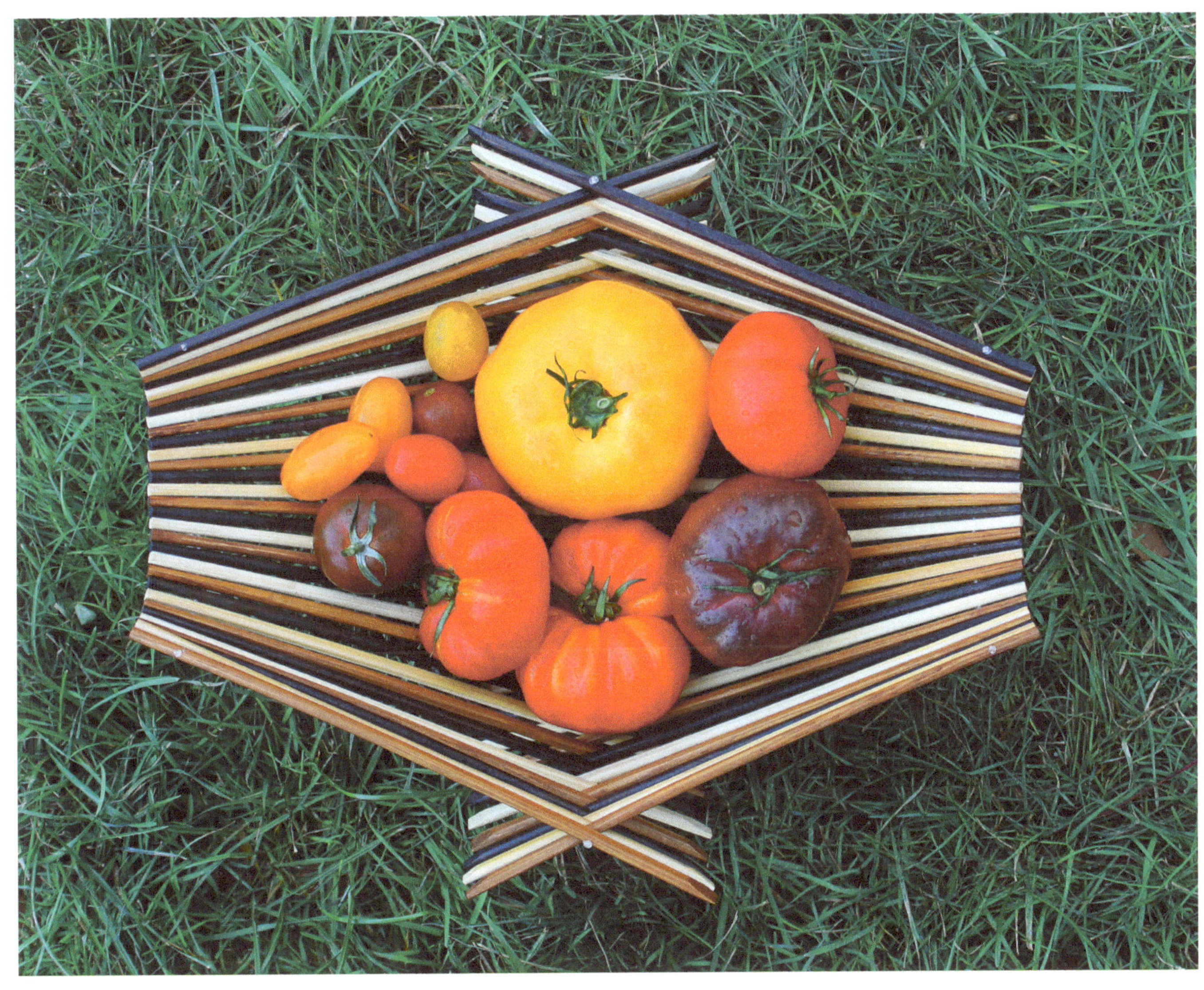

PEARS

CHEF DI'S TIP

Pears are one of my favorite fruits, mainly because they are in season nearly all year round. As a newbie into the diabetic world, picking the right fruit was a tough one for me. Of course, I had to decipher the time of day to eat fruit, and that was a little tricky too! Gone are the mornings where I could grab a bowl of mixed fruit and a muffin, or even fruit and a yogurt.

I usually eat pears alone or slice them into small wedges and add them to a gorgeous bowl of baby greens, chive vinaigrette, sliced grilled chicken, and lavender goat cheese. The best thing about pears is there are ten varieties, and each has its own distinct sweet and tangy flavor. The textures are so different too, from Seckel to Bosc to Asian and more. Have fun!

TANYA'S HEALTH BENEFITS

√ Excellent source of vitamin C, potassium, and fiber.
√ One medium-sized pear contains 6 grams of fiber.
√ Antioxidants found in pears and particularly pear skin may help increase insulin sensitivity in the body - critical in the prevention of Type 2 Diabetes.
√ May help prevent kidney stones.
√ A study examining apple and pear consumption found the combination of both reduced the risk of Type 2 Diabetes by 18%.

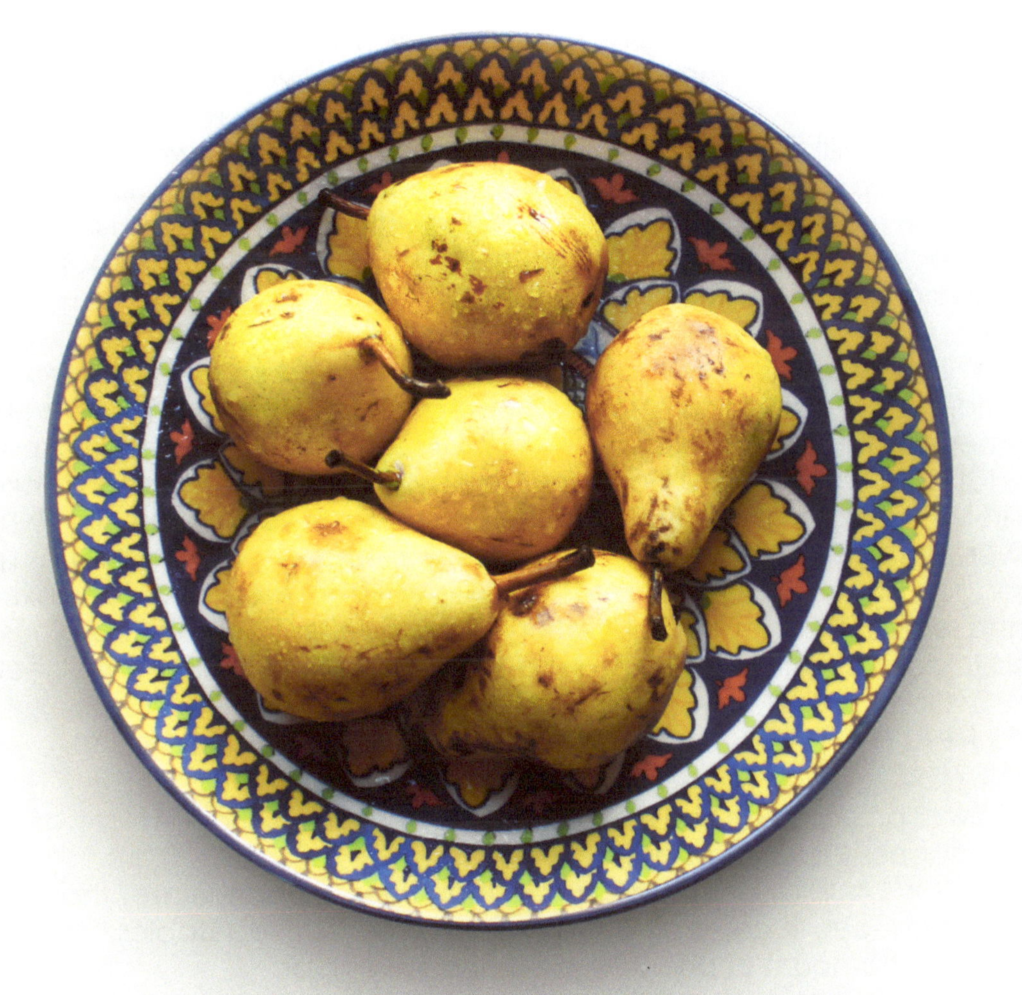

CAULIFLOWER

CHEF DI'S TIP

Isn't it funny how you were never exposed to certain types of vegetables as a child but now love them as an adult? I am not sure why my mom didn't cook cauliflower, but as an adult, I eat it all the time! I like to roast most of my vegetables, especially cauliflower. I learned a great recipe from New York Time's, Chef Julia Moskin. She puts the whole head of cauliflower, seasoned a little on the heavy side with extra virgin olive oil and salt and pepper, then roasts it for one to two hours at 375°F. She even bastes the cauliflower with more olive oil throughout the roasting process. What happens with this method, is you get this amazing crust on the bottom, which is simply out of this world. To serve it, you carve it into wedges and plate.

I love to cut my cauliflower into florets and rub it with a mixture of extra virgin olive oil, turmeric, cumin, and curry. After it is roasted and toasted, I add some chopped mint, pomegranate, and pistachios. This is a recipe I learned from Chef Andres at the Hudson Hotel. As a chef, I love being inspired by other chefs, and then make my own twist on it. My amazing niece, Bia, who lives in Brazil, is a vegetarian chef who roasts her cauliflower with curry and pimenta-do-reino (pink pepper), which is not as spicy as our black pepper. Bia will then make a tofu crema with roasted garlic, tofu, extra virgin olive oil, and lemon. This great combination of ingredients is insanely delicious! Whenever I can find tri-color cauliflower heads, I use them for color. It makes a gorgeous dish.

TANYA'S HEALTH BENEFITS

√ Cauliflower packs a nutritious punch of vitamins A and C and folate as well as miner als like magnesium and potassium.

√ In particular, cauliflower contains a phytonutrient (glucosinolate) that is known to help prevent cancer. In comparison to other cruciferous vegetables, cauliflower contains the highest amount of phenolic acid and flavonoids.

√ Cauliflower has less vitamin K than many of the other members of the cruciferous vegetable family, especially in comparison to the green leafy vegetables, which are a better choice if you are at risk for blood clots.

√ Steam, sauté, roast, and bake cruciferous vegetables for the most benefits. Avoid boiling as the boiling process reduces phytonutrient content significantly.

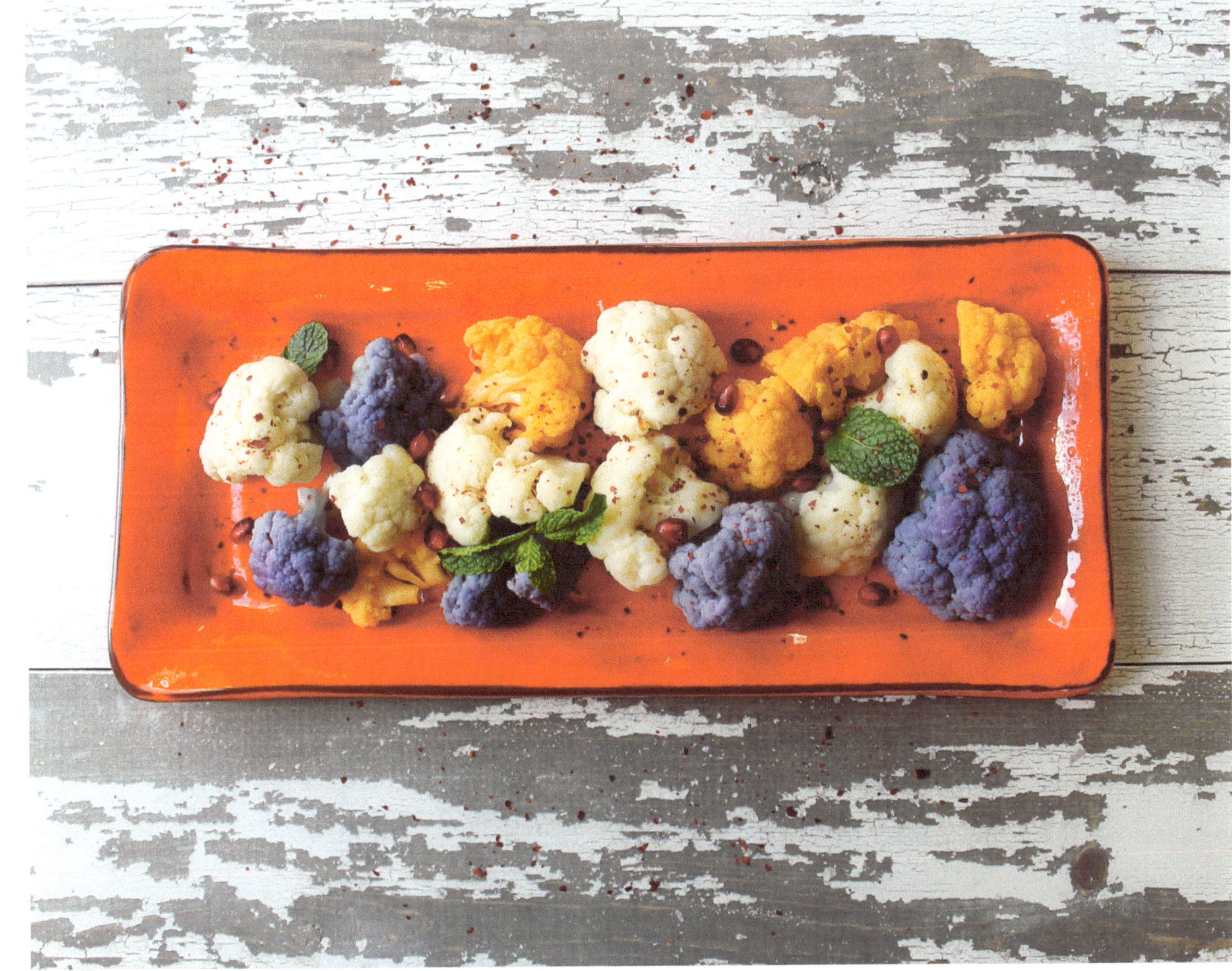

GARLIC

CHEF DI'S TIP

I once had a lovely neighbor tell me she hates the smell of garlic. I thought, "Oh no, we are in trouble. I love garlic and use it in nearly everything I make!" In fact, I could not imagine having an allergy to garlic. It is a wonderful addition to every dish. When I started to buy garlic bulbs from the Farmer's Market, I learned how much better it was than the garlic I bought at the local supermarkets. It lost that harsh back-of-the-throat-flavor and the fresh right-from-the-ground garlic bulb adds a gentle sweetness to all the dishes I cook. When I toast it and sprinkle it on salads or any type of meal, the crunchy texture, and full body flavor transforms the food. My mom loves garlic too. She microwaves the whole bulb for a few seconds, and that small amount of heat allows her to peel the skins right off. Mom said when she does this, it helps her digestion process!

TANYA'S HEALTH BENEFITS

√ Reduces both systolic and diastolic blood pressure.
√ Shown to improve cholesterol, LDL cholesterol, and HDL cholesterol numbers.
√ Allicin is a known bioactive compound in garlic, activated when garlic is chopped or crushed. Studies have shown garlic supplements high in allicin help reduce blood sugar and prevent Type 2 Diabetes.
√ May have been fed to athletes in the earliest Olympic games to increase stamina in ancient Greece.

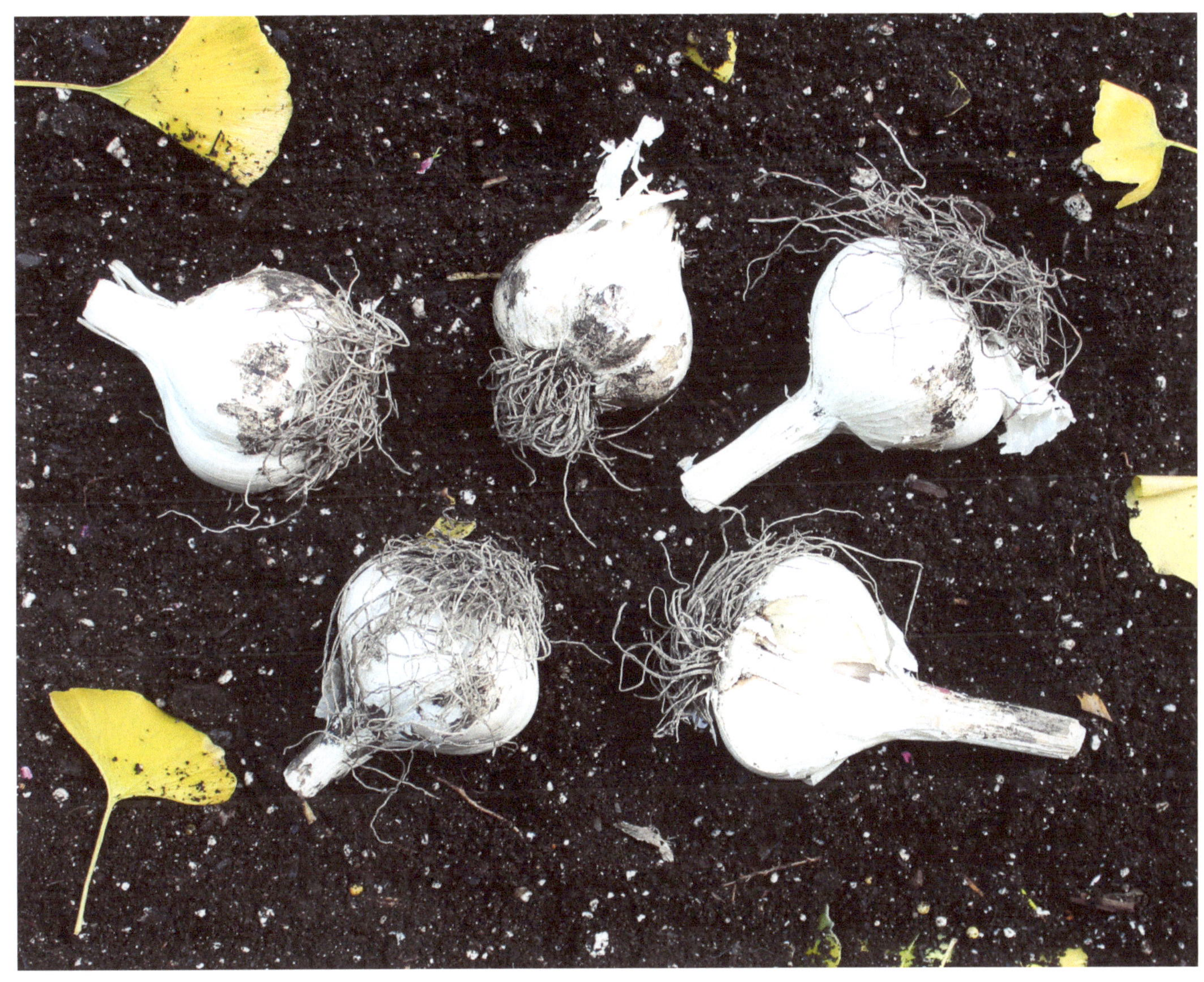

NUTS & SEEDS

CHEF DI'S TIP

This is another food item I cannot live without. I buy a variety of nuts and seeds, mix them all together, and have them in the kitchen at all times. I use nuts and seeds in so many dishes from salads to soup garnishes to main dishes. I always carry them in my snack bag. I like them raw, so I do not toast or roast them, but they can be prepared that way too. I also was told by another one of my nutritionists to soak them overnight so they can be digested easier. Again, I do not do it myself, but I have heard people can digest nuts better if they are soaked. I love all nuts and seeds (except for peanuts). My favorite mix lately is a combination of pecans, almonds, walnuts, hazelnuts, cashews, pumpkin, and sunflower seeds.

TANYA'S HEALTH BENEFITS

√ 1/4 cup of sunflower seeds provides 82% of your daily value of vitamin E vital for skin health.

√ Excellent source of omega-3 fatty acids, fiber, magnesium.

√ The omega-3 fatty acids in sunflower seeds can help prevent depression and anxiety, protect skin from sun damage, and improve heart health.

√ Pumpkin seeds, especially the unshelled ones, are an excellent source of zinc.

√ Pumpkin seeds are one of the best sources of the mineral manganese. While most are not deficient, an association has been found between deficiency of manganese and both diabetes and renal dysfunction.

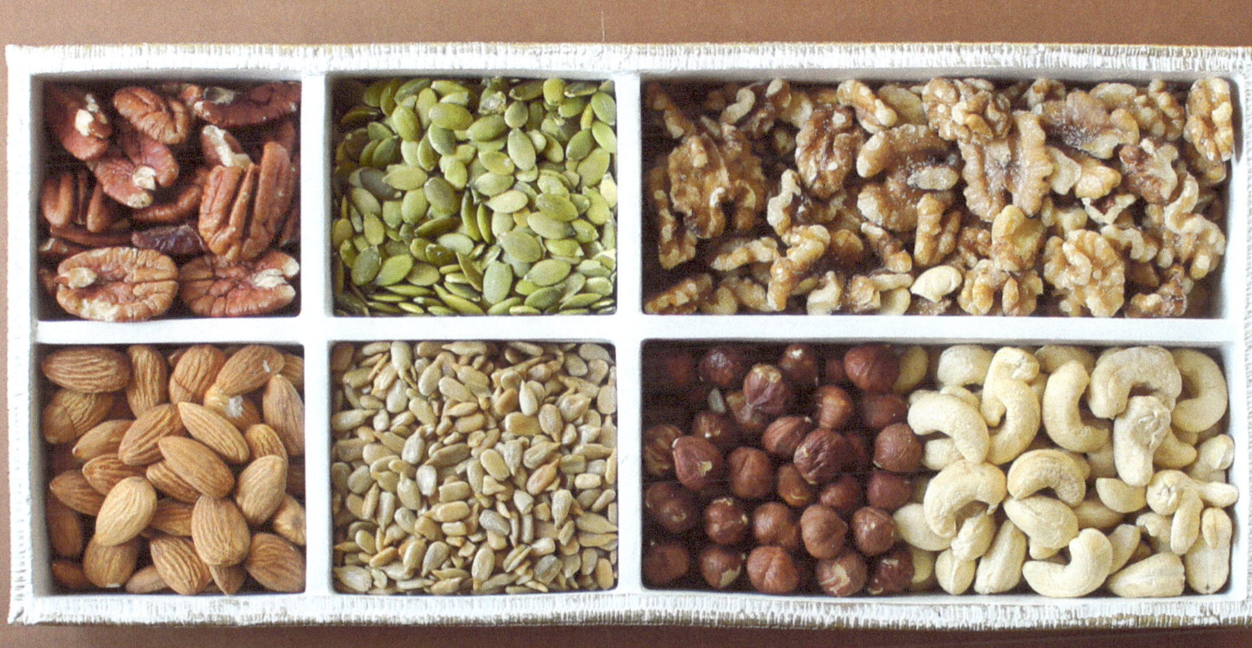
XOXO

RESOURCES & SOURCES

TANYA'S LIST

Sugar/Insulin
https://www.ncbi.nlm.nih.gov/pmc/articles/PMC5174139/?

Walnuts and Melatonin
Nutrients (ISSN 2072-6643; CODEN: NUTRHU) is a peer-reviewed open access journal of human nutrition published monthly online by MDPI. https://www.ncbi.nlm.nih.gov/pmc/articles/PMC5409706/
https://www.ncbi.nlm.nih.gov/pmc/articles/PMC5133084/
https://www.ncbi.nlm.nih.gov/pmc/articles/PMC5174139/
https://www.ncbi.nlm.nih.gov/pmc/articles/PMC5174149/
https://www.ncbi.nlm.nih.gov/pubmed/26376619

Selenium
Institute of Medicine. Food and Nutrition Board. Dietary Reference Intakes for Vitamin C, Vitamin E, Selenium, and Carotenoids. National Academies Press. Washington, DC, 2000.
PMID: 25077263
www.ncbi.nlm.nih.gov/pubmed/25077263.

USDA nutrient database

Carrots and turning orange
https://www.tandfonline.com/doi/abs/10.3109/09637486.2010.511164
Carrots – lutein – eye health
https://bjo.bmj.com/content/101/5/551 quercetin
https://www.ncbi.nlm.nih.gov/pmc/articles/PMC4808895/ red sorrel
https://scialert.net/fulltext/?doi=rjphyto.2008.69.76
https://www.webmd.com/vitamins/ai/ingredientmono-718/sorrel
https://www.ncbi.nlm.nih.gov/pmc/articles/PMC4745323/
https://www.organicfacts.net/health-benefits/herbs-and-spices/sorrel.html

Meyer Lemons
https://www.npr.org/templates/story/story.php?storyId=100778147

Radish
http://www.aicr.org/press/health-features/health-talk/2014/oct14/cruciferous-vegetables-health-benefits.html

Red Cabbage
https://nutritiondata.self.com/facts/vegetables-and-vegetable-products/2373/2
http://www.whfoods.com/genpage.php?tname=foodspice&dbid=19
Bacchetti T, Tullii D, Masciangelo S, et al. Effect of black and red cabbage on plasma carotenoid levels, lipid profile, and oxidized low-density lipoprotein. Journal of Functional Foods, Volume 8, May 2014, pages 128-137.

Pumpkin seeds, manganese, blood sugar control
https://www.ncbi.nlm.nih.gov/pmc/articles/PMC3973834/

Coconuts - https://www.ncbi.nlm.nih.gov/pmc/articles/PMC4671521/ https://www.ncbi.nlm.nih.gov/pmc/articles/PMC4892314/ https://www.ncbi.nlm.nih.gov/pmc/articles/PMC6255029/

Hemp seeds and chia seeds
https://www.hsph.harvard.edu/nutritionsource/food-features/chia-seeds/

Watercress/Brussel sprouts
https://www.mdpi.com/1420-3049/23/5/1139/htm

Dandelion greens
https://www.ars.usda.gov/plains-area/gfnd/gfhnrc/docs/news-2013/dark-green-leafy-vegetables/

Brussel sprouts
https://www.ncbi.nlm.nih.gov/pmc/articles/PMC4812465/

Pumpkin seeds
https://www.tandfonline.com/doi/abs/10.1080/10408398.2011.635816?journalCode=bfsn20
https://www.tandfonline.com/doi/abs/10.1080/10408398.2011.635816?journalCode=bfsn20

Pecans - https://www.ncbi.nlm.nih.gov/pmc/articles/PMC5872757/
https://www.ncbi.nlm.nih.gov/pubmed/10719404

Hazelnuts
https://www.ncbi.nlm.nih.gov/pmc/articles/PMC5188407/

Mushrooms
https://www.ncbi.nlm.nih.gov/pubmed/15630237
https://ndb.nal.usda.gov/ndb/foods/show/11987?fgcd=&manu=&format=Full&count=&max=25&offset=&sort=default&order=asc&qlookup=mushroom&ds=SR&qt=&qp=&qa-=&qn=&q=&ing=

Iron
https://ods.od.nih.gov/factsheets/Iron-HealthProfessional/

Potassium
https://ods.od.nih.gov/factsheets/Potassium-HealthProfessional/

Zinc - https://ods.od.nih.gov/factsheets/Zinc-HealthProfessional/

Figs - https://www.ncbi.nlm.nih.gov/pubmed/25017517 https://healthyeating.sfgate.com/figs-body-1779.html
J Ethnopharmacol. 2018 Apr 6;215:210-232. doi: 10.1016/j.jep.2017.12.045. Epub 2018 Jan 3. A role of Ficus species in the management of diabetes mellitus: A review. Deepa P1, Sowndhararajan K2, Kim S3, Park SJ4.
https://www.sciencedirect.com/science/article/pii/S0378874117333688?via%3Dihub

Shungiku
http://www.namayasai.co.uk/Shungiku/Shungiku2.htm https://www.healwithfood.org/health-benefits/garland-chrysanthemum-leaves.php

Nasturtium
https://www.ncbi.nlm.nih.gov/pmc/articles/PMC4307276/
https://ndb.nal.usda.gov/ndb/foods/show/302151?n1=%7BQv%3D1%7D&fgcd=&man=&lfacet=&count=&max=&sort=&qlookup=&offset=&format=Full&new=&measureby=&Qv=1&ds=&qt=&qp=&qa=&qn=&q=Watercress%2C+raw&ing=

Cherries
https://www.ncbi.nlm.nih.gov/pmc/articles/PMC5872786/ https://www.ncbi.nlm.nih.gov/pmc/articles/PMC3133468/

DIANA'S LIST

Peaches - https://www.grownyc.org/greenmarket/manhattan-union-square-m Red plate from https://www.williams-sonoma.com/

Avocado - Cutting Board from https://madmuseum.org/

Lemon and Lime - Cutting Board from https://www.homegoods.com/

Carrots - S&S.O Produce https://ssoproducefarms.com/

Persimmons - Bowl from https://www.williams-sonoma.com/

Tatsoi - Bowl from Artist Margaret Braun http://www.margaretbraun.com/

Mushrooms - Blue Oyster Cultivation, Bulich Farms, Gail's Farms (Union Square Farmers Market)

Cucumbers - Sanditas from https://www.surlatable.com/Blue bowl: https://www.williams-sonoma.com/

Turnips - https://www.windfallfarms.com/

Hemp & Chia - wooden holder: https://www.surlatable.com/

Radish - https://www.windfallfarms.com/ and http://www.norwichmeadowsfarm.com/ White Platter from Artist Margaret Braun http://www.margaretbraun.com/

Pomegranate - Purple platter https://www.laterrinedirect.com/

Figs - https://www.grownyc.org/greenmarket/manhattan-union-square-m Blue/yellow from https://www.williams-sonoma.com/ (garnish greens from http://www.twoguysfromwoodbridge.com/

Red Sorrel-http://www.twoguysfromwoodbridge.com/ Yellow Plate https://www.laterrinedirect.com/
Squash Blossoms - https://www.windfallfarms.com/. Platter – Artist Margaret Braun http://www.margaret-braun.com/

Mixed Greens - Greens from http://www.twoguysfromwoodbridge.com/ https://www.windfallfarms.com/. Plates: https://www.laterrinedirect.com/

Tomatoes: Wooden basket https://madmuseum.org/

Pears: https://www.grownyc.org/greenmarket/manhattan-union-square-m Blue/yellow bowl https://www.williams-sonoma.com/

Cauliflower: Orange platter https://www.laterrinedirect.com/ Nuts: Wooden box https://www.homegoods.com/

THANK YOU

Truthfully, it takes a village to create a book. I never thought I would be an author. Now all I can think about is the series of 8x8 booklets I want to create and continuing to be the storyteller I now know I was born to be! Whether it be my book or another author's book, I believe we can all learn a great deal about humanity from storytelling. I also feel it connects us more as a community and reminds us that we have many more similarities than we do differences. Our world coming together like this is truly my wish.

Gratitude is home for me. It is in my every breath. So here is a sliver of my thanks to all of those I love.

Miss Hailey: My girl! It all started with you that day in the shop. You were and will always be my true inspiration.
Tanya: Who knew you would start guiding me as a nutritionist and then end up writing the health benefits in my book? Your wise and calm vibes have balanced me in more ways than you will ever know.
Adam Woods of Publish Drive: My publisher and guide. I signed up for a Publish Drive self-publishing class with you at the Y, never knowing how profound an impact you would have in my life. We have quite a ride ahead of us, my friend!
Miss Angela: My editor. You came into my life at the final hour and saved the day. You had me at your email name @butterflyangels.
Chuck P: My Creative Director. You are my dear friend who keeps it real, and never says, "it's nice."
My love for you has no boundaries. My posse: You know who you are. My amazing friends who I adore with all my heart. You have seen me through the good, the bad, and the ugly, I would so not be here without all of you.
My family: You will always be the most important people in my life. Forever love.
My teachers: There are too many to list but here are a few: Rebekah Boruki, Elena Brower, Gabby Bernstein, Allan Lokos, Sharon Salzberg, Pilar Jennings, Susie Brown, Shannon Algeo, Lora Krulak, and Laurie Gerber. You are the people who helped me clear the path and bring me to today. My bucket of gratitude overflows for you.
My love: My one and only, Billy. It is YOU who stood by me and always believed in me. Even when the words were not heard, they were always felt.

With gratitude and grace,

Di xox

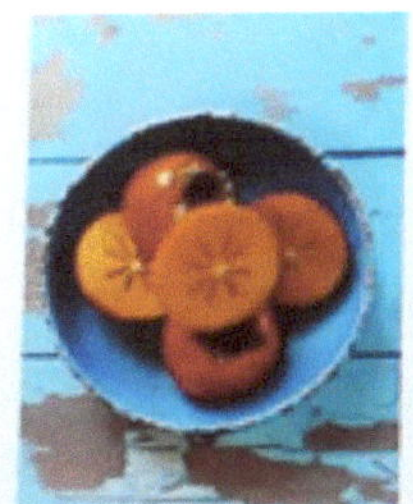

CARROTS

CHEF DI'S TIPS

TANYA'S HEALTH BENEFITS

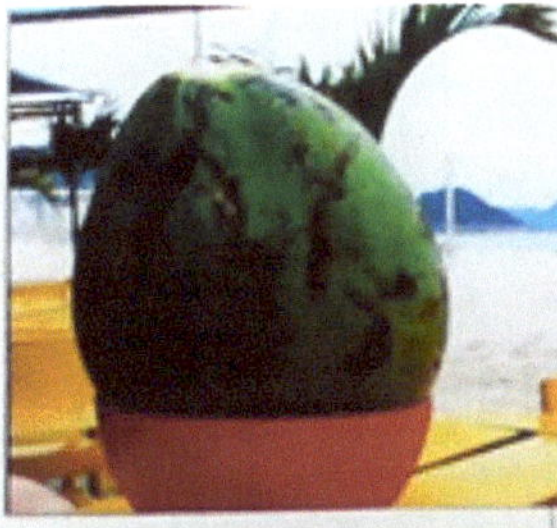

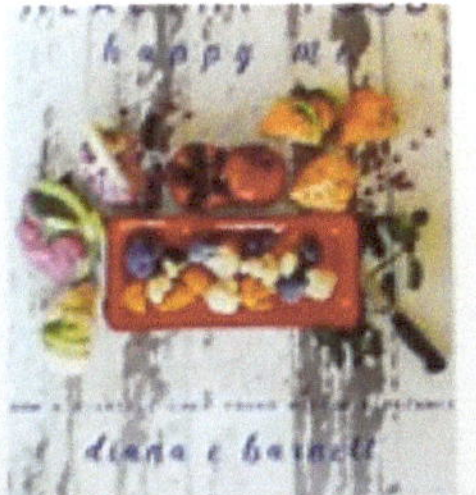

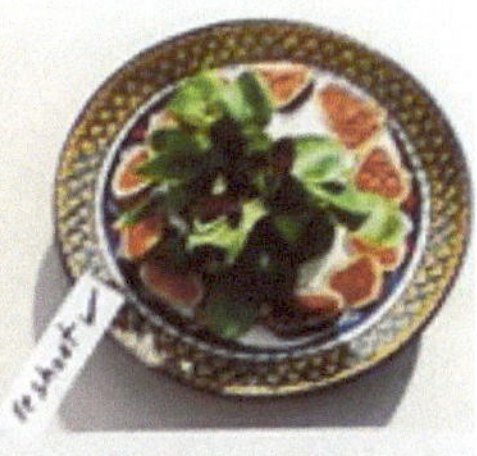

EGGS

CHEF DI'S TIPS

TANYA'S HEALTH BENEFITS

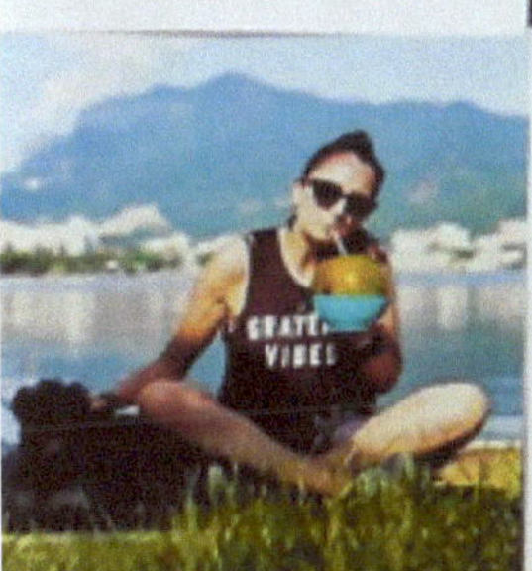

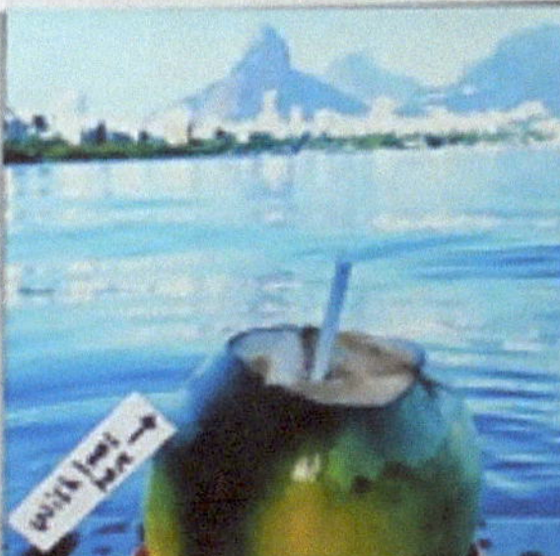

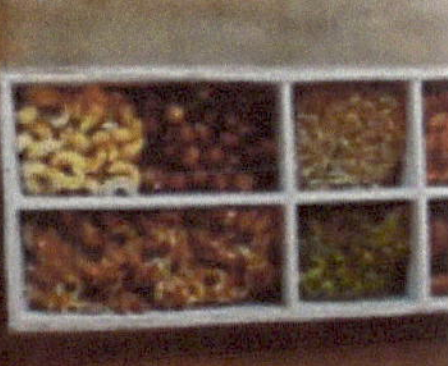

CAULIFLOWER

CHEF DI'S TIPS

TANYA'S HEALTH BENEFITS

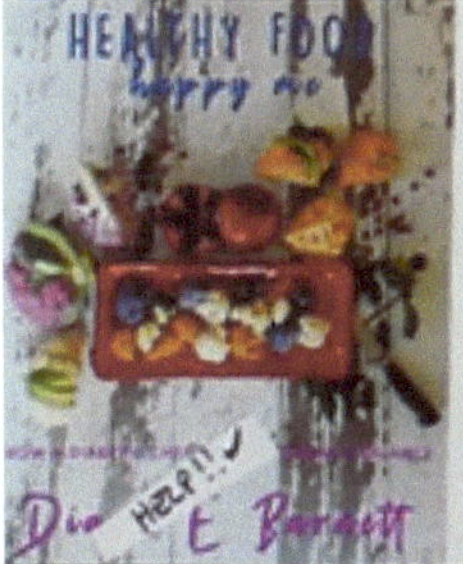

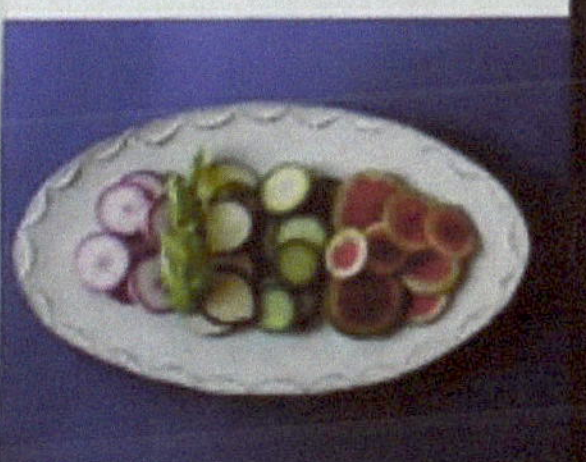

GARLIC

CHEF DI'S TIPS

TANYA'S HEALTH BENEFITS

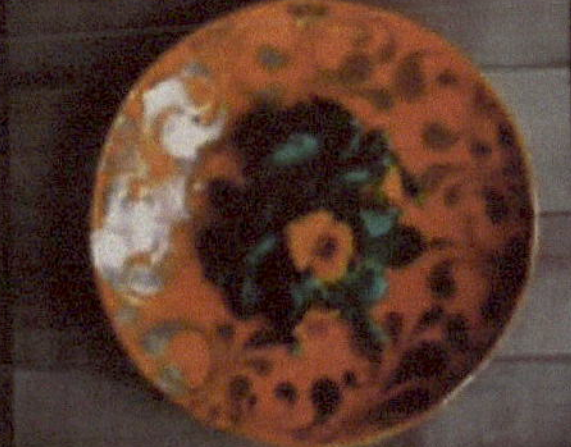

AVOCADOS

CHEF DI'S TIPS

TANYA'S HEALTH BENEFITS

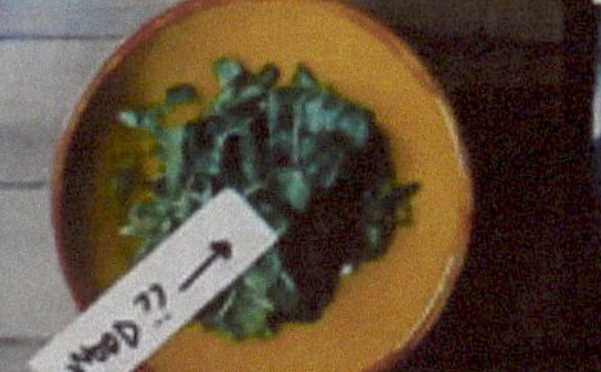

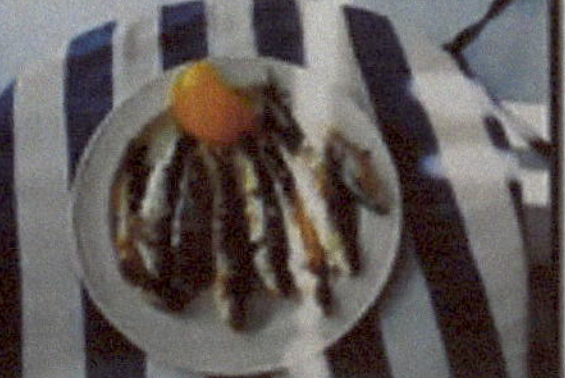

CUCUMBERS

CHEF DI'S TIPS

TANYA'S HEALTH BENEFITS

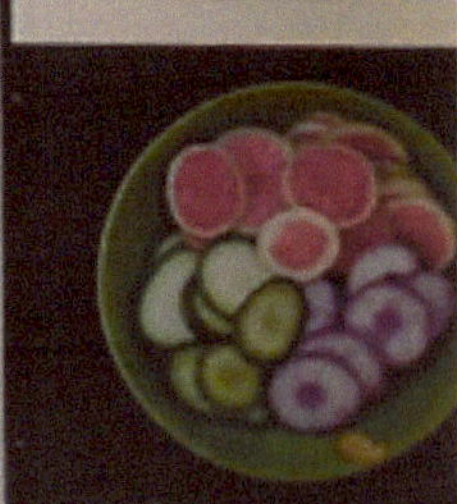

CPSIA information can be obtained
at www.ICGtesting.com
Printed in the USA
JSHW040326310123
36685JS00002B/3